NEW COMPLETE ZERO GRAVITY POINT RECIPE COOKBOOK 2024

(0) Point Complete Cookbook with, Fuss-free, Delicious & Easy to make Recipes for busy people Watching their Weight

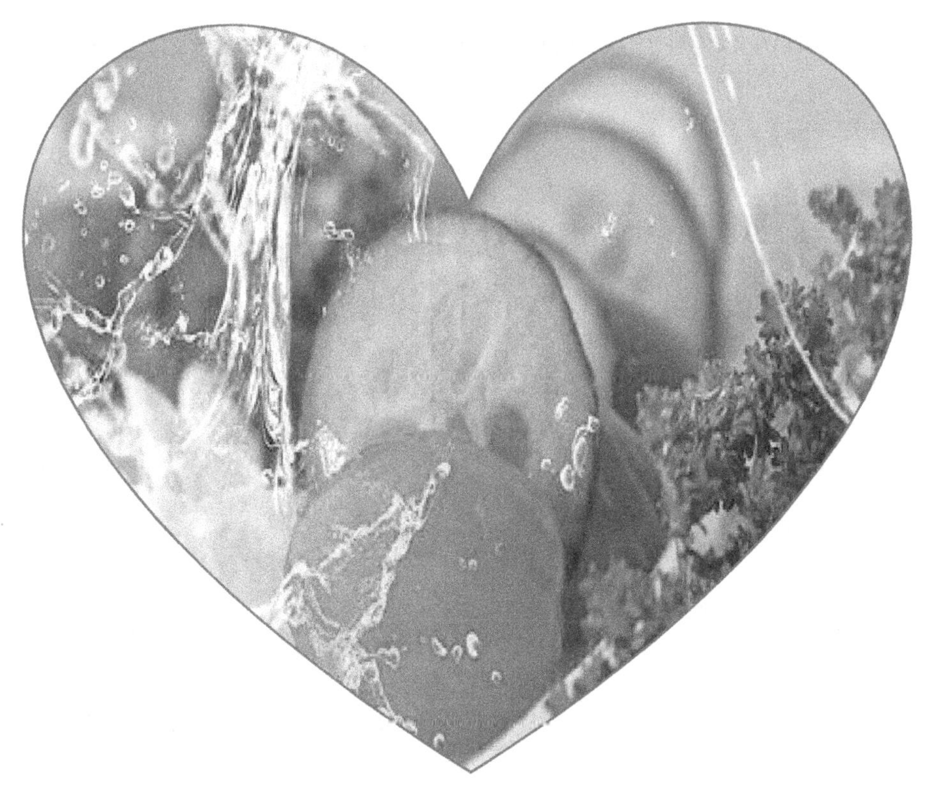

SARA JEFFREYS

Copyright © 2023 [SARA JEFFREYS]

This cookbook is a culinary creation designed for those embarking on a journey to wellness and mindful eating. The recipes contained within are crafted to align with the principles of the Zero Gravity Point program, providing a delightful array of dishes that are both nourishing and satisfying.

The author and publisher have invested considerable effort to ensure the accuracy and relevance of the information presented. However, it is important to note that this cookbook is not a substitute for professional medical advice. Readers are encouraged to consult with a qualified healthcare professional or a registered dietitian for personalized guidance based on their unique health circumstances

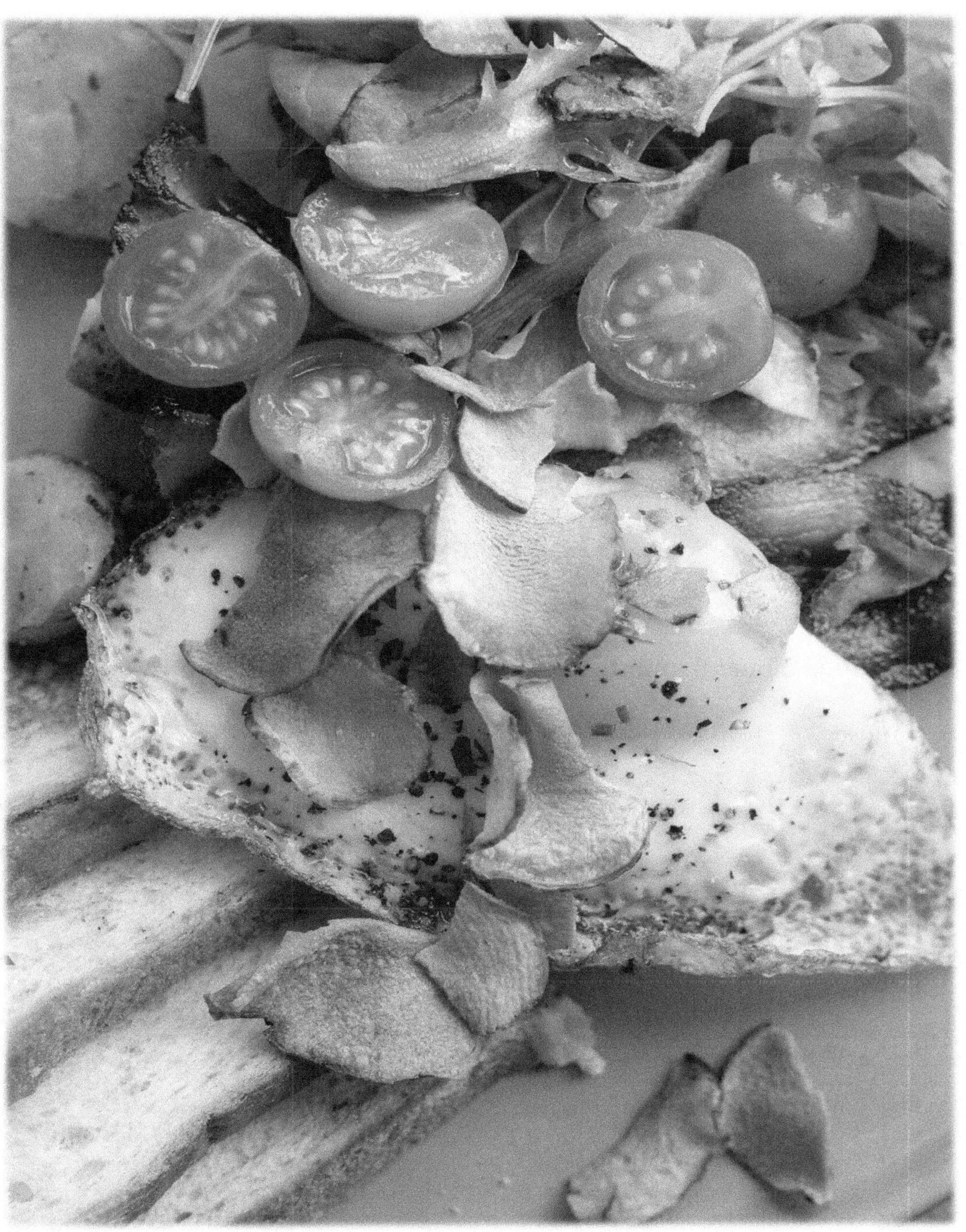

Z-P BREAKFAST RECIPES

01

Greek Goddess Smoothie

Preparation Time: 5 minutes

Servings: 2

Ingredients:

- 2 cups fresh spinach
- 1 ripe banana
- 1 cup Greek yogurt
- 1 cup almond milk
- 1 tablespoon honey (opt)
- 2 tablespoons chia seeds

Instructions:

- Combine Ingredients: In a blender, add spinach, banana, Greek yogurt, almond milk, and honey (if using).
- Blend Until Smooth: Blend the items until you achieve a smooth consistency.
- Serve: Pour the juice into cups and add chia seeds on top before serving.

Nutritional Value (Per Serving)::

Calories: 180 | Protein: 12g | Carbohydrates: 25g | Fat: 4g | Fiber: 6g

Health Benefits and Nutritional Insights:

1. Zero-Point Ingredients: This smoothie boasts zero-point ingredients according to the Weight Watching system, making it a great addition to a balanced, low-calorie meal plan.

2. High Nutrient Density: Spinach provides essential vitamins and minerals, including vitamin K, vitamin A, folate, and iron. Bananas offer potassium and natural sweetness, while Greek yogurt contributes protein and probiotics for gut health.

3. **Omega-3 Boost:** Chia seeds are a source of omega-3 fatty acids, fiber, and antioxidants, aiding in digestion and promoting heart health.

4. Satiety and Energy: With its blend of protein, healthy fats, and fiber, this smoothie offers sustained energy and keeps you feeling full throughout the morning, making it an ideal choice for breakfast.

Avocado Toast with Poached Egg

Preparation Time: 15 minutes

Servings: 2

Ingredients:

- 2 slices whole grain bread
- 1 ripe avocado
- 2 poached eggs
- 1 cup cherry tomatoes, halved
- Chili flakes (optional)

Instructions:

- Toast the bread slices.
- Mash ripe avocado and spread it evenly on the toasted bread.
- Top each slice with a poached egg.
- Arrange cherry tomato halves on top and sprinkle with chili flakes if desired.

Nutritional Value (Per Serving)::

Calories: 290, Protein: 12g,

Carbohydrates: 20g, Fat: 18g,

Fiber: 8g

Health Benefits and Nutritional Insights:

1. Heart-Healthy Fats: Avocado provides healthy monounsaturated fats, fiber, and various vitamins and minerals, promoting heart health and satiety.
2. Protein Power: Poached eggs offer high-quality protein and essential nutrients.
3. Antioxidant Boost: Cherry tomatoes are rich in antioxidants like lycopene, contributing to overall health and well-being.

Berry Chia Pudding

Preparation Time: 10 minutes (+overnight chilling)

Servings: 4

Ingredients:

- 1/2 cup chia seeds
- 2 cups almond milk
- 1 cup mixed berries (strawberries, blueberries, raspberries)
- 2 tablespoons honey
- Sliced nuts for garnish

Instructions:

- In a bowl, mix chia seeds and almond milk. Stir well and let it sit for 5 minutes. Stir again to avoid clumps.
- Gently fold in the mixed berries and honey.
- Cover the bowl and chill overnight or for at least 4 hours.
- Serve chilled, topped with sliced nuts.

Nutritional Value (Per Serving)::

Calories: 170 | Protein: 5g

Carbohydrates: 20g | Fat: 9g | Fiber: 10g

Health Benefits and Nutritional Insights:

- Omega-3 and Fiber: Chia seeds are a rich source of omega-3 fatty acids and dietary fiber, helping digestion and promoting heart health.
- Antioxidant-Rich Berries: Mixed berries offer a wealth of antioxidants, vitamins, and minerals, boosting system function and lowering inflammation.

Banana Walnut Overnight Oats

Preparation Time: 5 minutes (+overnight chilling)

Servings: 2

Ingredients:

- 1 cup rolled oats
- 1 cup almond milk
- 1 ripe banana, mashed
- 1/4 cup chopped walnuts
- Maple syrup for drizzling (optional)

Instructions:

- In a jar or bowl, mix rolled oats and almond milk.
- Add mashed banana and chopped walnuts, stir well.
- Cover and refrigerate overnight.
- Serve chilled, drizzle with maple syrup if wanted.

Nutritional Value (Per Serving)::

Calories: 280, Protein: 7g, Carbohydrates: 42g, Fat: 10g, Fiber: 7g

Health Benefits and Nutritional Insights:

1. Fiber and Potassium: Bananas offer potassium, helping in muscle function, along with fiber for better absorption.
2. Omega-3s from Walnuts: Walnuts add omega-3 fatty acids and vitamins, helping heart health.

Vegetable Omelette Wraps

Preparation Time: 15 minutes

Servings: 2

Ingredients:

- 4 eggs
- 1/2 cup diced bell peppers
- 1 cup chopped spinach
- 1/2 cup chopped tomatoes
- 1/4 cup low-fat cheese (optional)
- 2 whole grain wraps

Instructions:

- Beat eggs in a bowl and add pepper and salt to taste.
- In a non-stick pan, sauté bell peppers, spinach, and tomatoes until softened.
- Pour beaten eggs over the sautéed veggies and cook until set.
- Sprinkle with cheese if using, then split the egg into two pieces.
- Place each piece in a whole grain wrap and fold it into a wrap.

Nutritional Value (Per Serving)::

Calories: 320, Protein: 20g, Carbohydrates: 24g, Fat: 15g, Fiber: 6g

Health Benefits and Nutritional Insights:

1. Protein and veggies: This dish offers a protein-rich breakfast with a mix of bright veggies, giving vitamins, minerals, and fiber.

Greek Yogurt Parfait

Preparation Time: 10 minutes

Servings: 2

Ingredients:

- 2 cups Greek yogurt

- One cup of mixed fresh berries, including of raspberries, blueberries, and strawberries

- 1/2 cup granola

- Honey for dripping (optional)

Instructions:

- In serving cups or bowls, add Greek yogurt, mixed berries, and granola.

- Layers should be repeated until the glasses are full.

- Drizzle honey on top if wanted.

Nutritional Value (Per Serving)::

- Calories: 280

- Protein: 20g

- Carbohydrates: 40g

- Fat: 5g

- Fiber: 6g

Health Benefits and Nutritional Insights:

1. Protein-Packed: Greek yogurt offers a substantial protein source, helping in muscle repair and satisfaction.

2. Antioxidants and Fiber: Berries offer antioxidants and fiber, boosting general health and helping digestion.

Smoked Salmon and Cream Cheese Bagel

Preparation Time: 10 minutes

Servings: 2

Ingredients:

- 2 whole grain bagels, sliced and toasted

- 4 tablespoons light cream cheese
- 100g smoked salmon
- 1/2 cup cucumber slices
- Fresh dill for garnish

Instructions:

- Spread light cream cheese on the toasted bread halves.
- Arrange a layer of smoked salmon over the cream cheese.
- Add cucumber slices over the salmon.
- Garnish with fresh dill.

Nutritional Value (Per Serving)::

Calories: 320, Protein: 20g, Carbohydrates: 35g, Fat: 12g, Fiber: 6g

Health Benefits and Nutritional Insights:

1. Omega-3s from Salmon: Smoked salmon offers heart-healthy omega-3 fatty acids.
2. Whole Grains and Protein: Whole grain bagels offer fiber while the mix of protein from salmon and cream cheese helps in satisfaction.

Fruit and Nut Butter Rice Cakes

Preparation Time: 5 minutes

Servings: 2

Ingredients:

- 4 rice cakes
- 4 tablespoons almond or peanut butter
- 1 ripe banana, sliced
- Mixed nuts (almonds, walnuts, etc.) for topping

Instructions:

- Spread almond or peanut butter evenly on each rice cake.
- Arrange banana slices on top of the nut butter.
- Sprinkle mixed nuts over the bananas.

Nutritional Value (Per Serving)::

- Calories: 280
- Protein: 7g
- Carbohydrates: 30g
- Fat: 16g
- Fiber: 4g

Health Benefits and Nutritional Insights:

1. Healthy Fats and Protein: Nut butter offers healthy fats and protein, helping in energy and satisfaction.
2. Fruit and Fiber: Bananas add fiber, vitamins, and minerals while rice cakes offer a gluten-free, low-calorie base.

Spinach and Feta Egg Cups

Preparation Time: 15 minutes

Servings: 4

Ingredients:

- 6 eggs
- 1 cup chopped spinach
- 1/2 cup crumbled feta cheese
- 1/2 cup chopped tomatoes
- Salt and pepper to taste

Instructions:

- Preheat the oven to 350°F (175°C). Grease a muffin pan.
- Beat the eggs and add salt and pepper to taste in a bowl.

- Add chopped spinach, feta cheese, and diced tomatoes to the beaten eggs, mix well.
- Evenly pour mixture into muffin pan.
- Bake for 12-15 minutes or until the egg cups are set.

Nutritional Value (Per Serving)::

Calories: 140, Protein: 10g, Carbohydrates: 3g, Fat: 10g, Fiber: 1g

Health Benefits and Nutritional Insights:

1. Protein and Calcium: Eggs and feta cheese provide a good amount of protein and calcium, boosting muscle and bone health.

2. Vegetables and Antioxidants: Spinach and tomatoes offer important vitamins, minerals, and antioxidants, adding to general well-being.

Cottage Cheese Pancakes

Preparation Time: 15 minutes

Servings: 2

Ingredients:

- 1 cup fat-free cottage cheese
- 1/2 cup rolled oats
- 2 eggs
- 1 teaspoon vanilla flavor
- Cooking spray or a little amount of oil

Instructions:

- Blend cottage cheese, rolled oats, eggs, and vanilla extract in a blender until smooth.
- Heat a non-stick pan over medium heat and lightly coat with cooking spray or oil.
- Pour small amounts of the pancake batter onto the pan to form pancakes.
- Cook for two to three minutes on each side, or until golden brown.

Nutritional Value (Per Serving)::

Calories: 220, Protein: 22g, Carbohydrates: 17g, Fat: 7g, Fiber: 2g

Health Benefits and Nutritional Insights:

1. High Protein: Cottage cheese is a great form of protein, helping in muscle repair and giving satisfaction.
2. Low-Calorie and Filling: These pancakes are low in calories but high in protein, making them a filling meal choice.

Mango Coconut Smoothie

Preparation Time: 5 minutes

Servings: 2

Ingredients:

- 1 mature mango, peeled and diced
- 1 cup coconut water
- Juice of 1 lime
- Handful of shredded coconut

Instructions:

- In a mixer, add chopped mango, coconut water, and lime juice.
- Blend until smooth and creamy.
- Serve in cups and top with shredded coconut.

Nutritional Value (Per Serving)::

Calories: 120, Protein: 1g, Carbohydrates: 30g, Fat: 1g, Fiber: 4g

Health Benefits and Nutritional Insights:

1. Vitamins and Minerals: Mangoes are rich in vitamins A and C, while coconut water offers fluids and hydration.
2. Fiber and Refreshment: This drink is not only hydrating but also offers a good amount of fiber, helping digestion and supporting general health.

Peanut Butter Banana Wrap

Preparation Time: 5 minutes

Servings: 2

Ingredients:

- 2 whole grain wraps
- 4 tablespoons peanut butter
- 2 ripe bananas, sliced
- A sprinkle of spice

Instructions:

- Spread peanut butter evenly on each whole grain wrap.
- Arrange banana slices on top of the peanut butter.
- Sprinkle a dash of cinnamon over the bananas.

- Roll the wraps and slice in half if wanted.

Nutritional Value (Per Serving)::

Calories: 320, Protein: 8g, Carbohydrates: 48g, Fat: 12g, Fiber: 8g

Health Benefits and Nutritional Insights:

1. Healthy Fats and Energy: Peanut butter offers healthy fats and protein, giving steady energy.
2. Potassium and Fiber: Bananas add potassium and fiber, boosting heart health and nutrition.

Egg and Veggie Breakfast Tacos

Preparation Time: 15 minutes

Servings: 2

Ingredients:

- 4 eggs
- 1/2 cup diced bell peppers
- 1 cup chopped spinach
- 1/2 cup chopped tomatoes
- Salt and pepper to taste
- 4 corn tortillas

Instructions:

- In a pan, sauté diced bell peppers, chopped spinach, and diced tomatoes until softened.
- In a different bowl, beat eggs and season with salt and pepper.
- Pour the beaten eggs into the pan with the sautéed veggies and mix until cooked.
- Warm the corn tortillas in a different pan or oven.

- Divide the egg and veggie mixture among the rolls and fold them into tacos.

Nutritional Value (Per Serving)::

Calories: 280, Protein: 14g, Carbohydrates: 25g, Fat: 12g, Fiber: 5g

Health Benefits and Nutritional Insights:

1. Protein and Veggies: This dish blends protein-rich eggs with a range of bright veggies, giving important nutrients and fiber.

Blueberry Almond Butter Toast

Preparation Time: 5 minutes

Servings: 2

Ingredients:

- 4 slices whole grain bread, toasted
- 4 tablespoons almond butter
- 1 cup fresh blueberries
- Honey for dripping (optional)

Instructions:

- Spread almond butter evenly on each warm slice of bread.
- Arrange fresh blueberries on top of the almond butter.
- Drizzle honey over the blueberries if wanted.

Nutritional Value (Per Serving)::

Calories: 290, Protein: 10g, Carbohydrates: 35g, Fat: 14g, Fiber: 6g

Health Benefits and Nutritional Insights:

1. **Healthy Fats and Antioxidants:** Almond butter offers healthy fats and protein, while blueberries provide antioxidants and vitamins, supporting general health.

Quinoa Breakfast Bowl

Preparation Time: 15 minutes

Servings: 2

Ingredients:

- 1 cup cooked quinoa
- 1/2 cup Greek yogurt
- 1 apple, diced
- 1/2 teaspoon cinnamon
- Handful of nuts (almonds, walnuts) for topping

Instructions:

- In a bowl, add cooked rice and Greek yogurt.
- Add diced apples on top of the yogurt.
- Sprinkle cinnamon over the apples and rice.
- Top with a handful of nuts.

Nutritional Value (Per Serving)::

Calories: 280; Protein: 12g; Carbohydrates: 40g; Fat: 8g; Fiber: 6g

Health Benefits and Nutritional Insights:

2. Protein and Fiber: Greek yogurt and rice provide protein and fiber, helping in satisfaction and digestion.
3. Vitamins and Minerals: Apples offer vitamins and enzymes, while nuts contribute healthy fats and extra nutrients.

Chickpea Flour Pancakes

Preparation Time: 15 minutes

Servings: 2

Ingredients:

- 1 cup chickpea flour
- 1 cup water
- 1/2 teaspoon baking powder
- 1/2 teaspoon ground turmeric
- Cooking spray or a little amount of oil

Instructions:

- In a mixing bowl, whisk together chickpea flour, water, baking powder, and ground turmeric until a smooth batter forms.
- Heat a non-stick pan over medium heat and lightly coat with cooking spray or oil.
- Pour small amounts of the batter onto the pan to make pancakes.
- Cook for two to three minutes on each side, or until golden brown.

Nutritional Value (Per Serving)::

Calories: 220, Protein: 10g, Carbohydrates: 30g Fat: 5g, Fiber: 6g

Health Benefits and Nutritional Insights:

1. Gluten-Free and Protein-Rich: Chickpea flour offers a gluten-free option with a good amount of protein and fiber.
2. Turmeric's Benefits: Ground turmeric offers anti-

inflammatory benefits and vitamins.

Veggie Breakfast Burrito

Preparation Time: 15 minutes

Servings: 2

Ingredients:

- 4 eggs
- 1/2 cup sliced mushrooms
- 1 cup chopped spinach
- 1/4 cup diced onions
- 1/2 cup chopped tomatoes
- 2 whole grain tortillas

Instructions:

- In a pan, sauté sliced mushrooms, chopped spinach, diced onions, and diced tomatoes until softened.
- In a bowl, beat eggs and pour them into the pan with the sautéed veggies.
- Cook until the eggs are set and mix them with the veggies.
- Warm the whole grain tortillas in a different pan or oven.
- Divide the egg and veggie filling between the rolls and fold them into burritos.

Nutritional Value (Per Serving)::

Calories: 320, Protein: 16g, Carbohydrates: 30g. Fat: 15g, Fiber: 8g

Health Benefits and Nutritional Insights:

1. Vegetable Power: This burrito offers a mix of bright vegetables, giving important vitamins, minerals, and fiber.

2. Protein Boost: Eggs add high-quality protein, helping in muscle repair and satisfaction.

Apple Cinnamon Overnight Chia Pudding

Preparation Time: 10 minutes (+overnight chilling)

Servings: 2

Ingredients:

- 1/4 cup chia seeds
- 1 1/2 cups unsweetened almond milk
- 1 apple, diced
- 1 teaspoon cinnamon
- Honey or maple syrup for sweetness (optional)

Instructions:

- In a bowl or jar, mix chia seeds and almond milk. After giving it a good stir, wait five minutes. Stir again to avoid clumps.
- Add diced apple and cinnamon to the chia blend. You can add honey or maple syrup , only if you want to. Cover the bowl or jar and chill overnight or for at least 4 hours.
- Serve cool.

Nutritional Value (Per Serving)::

Calories: 200, Protein: 6g, Carbohydrates: 28g. Fat: 8g, Fiber: 12g

Health Benefits and Nutritional Insights:

1. Fiber and Vitamins: Apples provide fiber and various

vitamins, while chia seeds offer omega-3 fatty acids and extra fiber.

2. Cinnamon's Benefits: Cinnamon may aid in regulating blood sugar levels and adds a delicious taste.

Turmeric Scrambled Tofu

Preparation Time: 10 minutes

Servings: 2

Ingredients:

- 1 block firm tofu, broken
- 1/2 teaspoon ground turmeric
- 1/2 cup diced bell peppers
- 1/4 cup diced onions
- 1 cup chopped spinach
- Salt and pepper to taste

Instructions:

- In a non-stick pan, sauté diced bell peppers, onions, and chopped spinach until softened.
- Add broken tofu to the pan and sprinkle with ground turmeric. Stir well to blend.
- Cook for 5-7 minutes until the tofu is cooked through and slightly golden.
- Season with salt and pepper to taste.

Nutritional Value (Per Serving)::

Calories: 180, Protein: 16g, Carbohydrates: 8g, Fat: 10g, Fiber: 3g

Health Benefits and Nutritional Insights:

1. Plant-Based Protein: Tofu offers a plant-based protein source, while ginger provides anti-inflammatory qualities and vitamins.
2. Vegetables and Fiber: Bell peppers, onions, and spinach add important nutrients and fiber to the dish.

Coconut Mango Smoothie

Preparation Time: 5 minutes

Servings: 2

Ingredients:

- 1 ripe mango, peeled and diced
- 1 cup coconut water
- Juice of 1 lime
- Handful of shredded coconut

Instructions:

- In a blender, combine diced mango, coconut water, and lime juice.
- Blend until smooth and creamy.
- Serve in glasses and garnish with shredded coconut.

Nutritional Value (Per Serving)::

Calories: 120, Protein: 1g, Carbohydrates: 30g, Fat: 1g, Fiber: 4g

Health Benefits and Nutritional Insights:

1. Vitamins and Minerals: Mangoes are rich in vitamins A and C, while coconut water provides electrolytes and hydration.
2. Fiber and Refreshment: This smoothie is not only hydrating

but also offers a good dose of
fiber, aiding digestion and
supporting overall health.

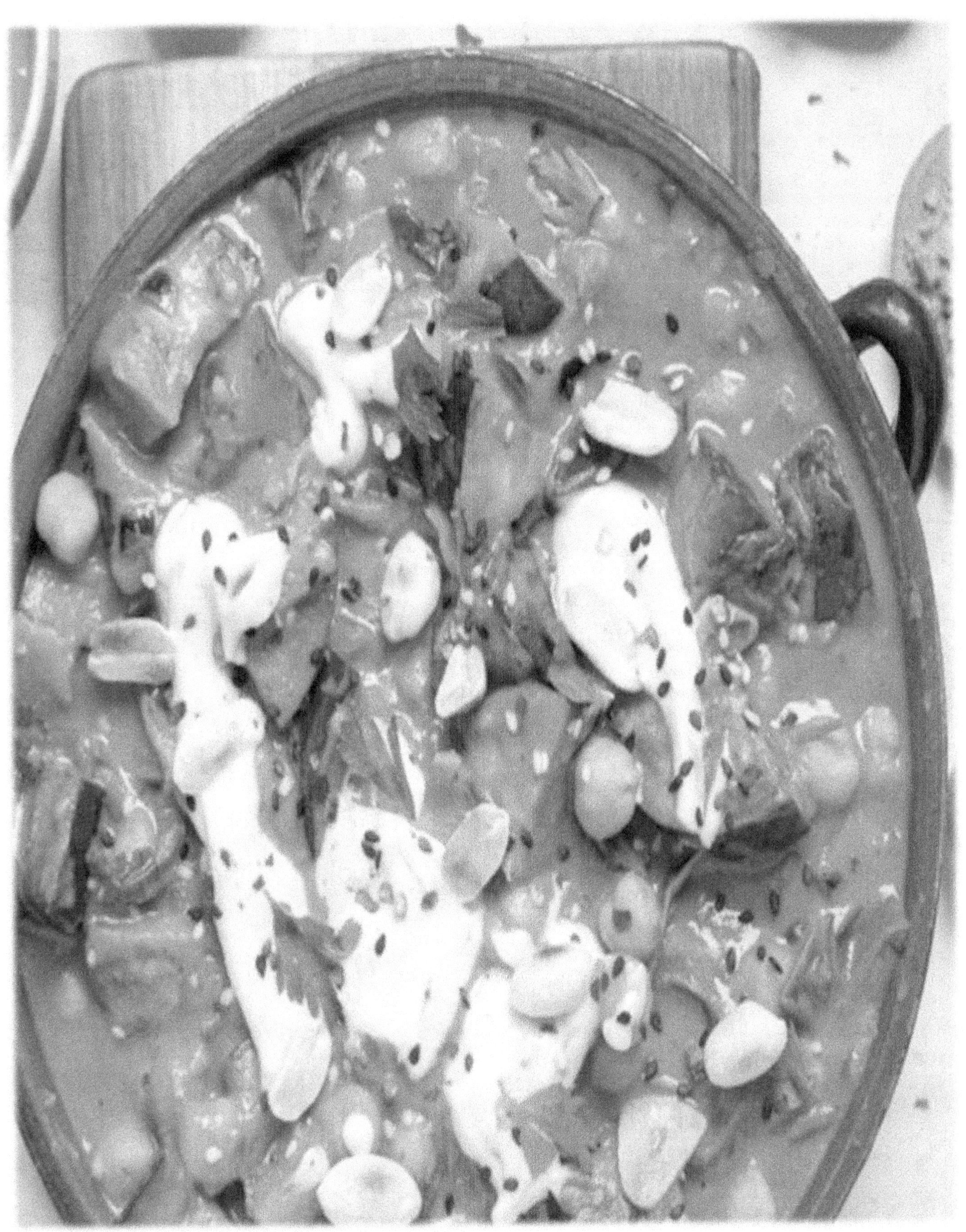

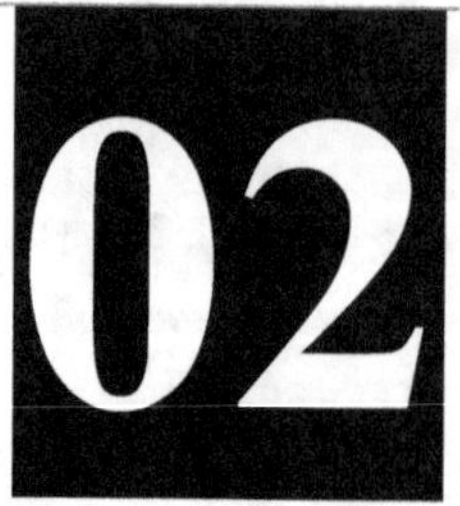

Chicken salad on the grill with balsamic vinaigrette:

Preparation Time: 15 minutes

Cook Time: 15 minutes (for frying chicken)

Servings: For 4 people

Ingredients:

- 1 pound of chicken breasts without bones or skin
- lettuce, spinach, and arugula mixed together in a salad bag.
- Cherry tomatoes, split
- Cucumbers, sliced
- Red onions, thinly sliced
- Balsamic vinegar sauce (zero-point or low-point choice)
- Salt and pepper to taste

Instructions:

- Season chicken breasts with salt and pepper.
- Grill the chicken until fully cooked, approximately 7-8 minutes per side.
- Take a few minutes to let the chicken rest before cutting it into strips.

- In a big bowl, mix salad leaves, cherry tomatoes, cucumbers, and red onions.
- Top the salad with grilled chicken strips.
- Drizzle balsamic dressing over the salad.
- Toss gently to mix.

Nutritional Value (per serve):

(Note: Nutritional values may change based on specific products and serving sizes.)

Calories: 250, Protein: 25g, Carbohydrates: 10g Fat: 12g, Fiber: 4g

Health Benefits:

1. High protein intake benefits muscle strength and satisfaction.
2. Low-calorie and nutrient-dense salad veggies provide vitamins and minerals.
3. Balsamic dressing gives taste without extra calories.
4. Vegetables add fiber and vitamins.

Vegetarian Quinoa Bowl with Roasted Vegetables:

Preparation Time: 20 minutes

Boiling Time: 25 minutes (for baking veggies and boiling rice)

Servings: 3

Ingredients:

- 1 cup quinoa, rinsed
- 2 cups mixed veggies (such as bell peppers, zucchini, cherry tomatoes)

- 1 tablespoon olive oil

- 1 teaspoon dried herbs (rosemary, thyme, or oregano)

- Salt and pepper to taste

- Feta cheese, crumbled (optional)

- Balsamic glaze (zero-point or low-point choice)

Instructions:

- Preheat the oven to 400°F (200°C).

- Toss mixed veggies with olive oil, chopped herbs, salt, and pepper.

- Roast the veggies on a baking sheet for 20-25 minutes or until golden.

- While the veggies are baking, cook quinoa according to package directions.

- In a bowl, combine the rice and roasted veggies.

- Top with chopped feta cheese if wanted.

- Drizzle with balsamic sauce before serving.

Nutritional Value:

(Note: Nutritional values may change based on specific products and serving sizes.)

Calories: 300 per serve, Protein: 10g, Carbohydrates: 50g, Fat: 8g, Fiber: 8g

Health Benefits:

1. Quinoa is a full energy source.
2. Colorful veggies provide a range of vitamins and minerals.
3. Olive oil adds healthy monounsaturated fats.
4. Feta cheese adds calcium and taste.

Zucchini Noodles with Pesto and Cherry Tomatoes:

Preparation Time:15 minutes.

Cooking Time: 5 minutes (for sautéing zucchini noodles)

Servings:2 cups

Ingredients:

- 2 large zucchinis, spiralized into noodles
- 1 cup cherry tomatoes, sliced
- 1/4 cup fresh basil leaves
- 2 tablespoons pine nuts
- 1 clove garlic, minced
- 2 tablespoons healthy yeast (extra)2 tablespoons olive oil
- Salt and pepper to taste
- Lemon zest for garnish

Instructions:

- In a food processor, mix basil, pine nuts, garlic, nutritional yeast, olive oil, salt, and pepper. Blend until a smooth pesto is made.
- Heat a pan over medium heat and add zucchini noodles. Sauté for 3-5 minutes until just soft.
- Toss the cherry tomatoes into the pan for the last minute of cooking, just to warm them through.
- Remove the pan from heat and mix in the made pesto.
- Serve the zucchini noodles and cherry tomatoes in bowls.
- Garnish with lemon zest and extra basil if wanted.

Nutritional Value:

(Note: Nutritional values may change based on specific products and serving sizes.)

Calories: 180 per serve, Protein: 5g, Carbohydrates: 10g, Fat: 15g, Fiber: 4g

Health Benefits:

1. Zucchini noodles are a low-calorie and low-carb option to standard pasta.
2. Pesto offers healthy fats from olive oil and pine nuts.
3. Cherry tomatoes offer vitamins and antioxidants.
4. Nutritional yeast adds a cheesy taste without dairy.

Turkey Lettuce Wraps with Hummus:

Preparation Time: 20 minutes

Cooking Time: 10 minutes (for cooking ground turkey)

Servings: 4

Ingredients:

- 1 lb lean ground turkey
- 1 tablespoon olive oil
- 1 teaspoon crushed cumin
- 1 teaspoon chopped coriander
- Salt and pepper to taste
- Iceberg or Romaine lettuce leaves, washed and dried
- 1 cup cherry tomatoes, diced
- 1 cucumber, diced
- 1/2 red onion, roughly chopped
- Hummus (zero-point or low-point choice)
- Fresh parsley, chopped (for garnish)

Instructions:

- On medium-low heat, add olive oil to a pan. Add ground turkey and cook until cooked.
- Season the turkey with cumin, cilantro, salt, and pepper. Stir well to blend.
- Remove the pan from heat and let the turkey cool slightly.
- Assemble lettuce wraps by putting a spoonful of cooked turkey in each lettuce leaf.
- Top with diced cherry tomatoes, cucumber, and red onion.
- Drizzle with hummus and top with fresh parsley.

Nutritional Value:

(Note: Nutritional values may change based on specific products and serving sizes.)

Calories: 220 per serve, Protein: 25g, Carbohydrates: 10g, Fat: 10g, Fiber: 3g

Health Benefits:

1. Lean ground turkey is a high-protein, low-fat meat choice.
2. Lettuce wraps lower calorie intake compared to standard wraps.
3. Vegetables add vitamins, minerals, and fiber.
4. Hummus offers a smooth, tasty topping.

Greek Chickpea Salad:

Preparation Time: 15 minutes

Servings: 4

Ingredients:

- 2 cans (15 oz each) chickpeas, drained and washed
- 1 cup cherry tomatoes, sliced
- 1 cucumber, diced
- 1/2 red onion, roughly chopped
- 1/2 cup Kalamata olives, chopped
- 1/2 cup crumbled feta cheese (optional)
- 1/4 cup fresh parsley, chopped
- For the Dressing:

- 3 tablespoons extra virgin olive oil
- 2 tablespoons red wine vinegar
- 1 teaspoon dried oregano
- Salt and pepper to taste

Instructions:

- In a big bowl, mix beans, cherry tomatoes, cucumber, red onion, Kalamata olives, and possible feta cheese.
- In a small bowl, mix together olive oil, red wine vinegar, dried oregano, salt, and pepper to make the sauce.
- Give the salad a gentle toss to mix after adding the sauce.
- Sprinkle fresh parsley over the top before serving.

Nutritional Value:

(Note: Nutritional values may change based on specific products and serving sizes.)

Calories: 280 per serve, Protein: 11g, Carbohydrates: 35g, Fat: 12g, Fiber: 10g

Health Benefits:

1. Chickpeas provide plant-based energy and fiber.

2. The salad is rich in veggies, giving different vitamins and minerals.

3. Olive oil adds heart-healthy monounsaturated fats.

4. Kalamata olives add a tasty touch while offering healthy fats.

Spaghetti Squash Primavera:

Preparation Time: 15 minutes.

Cooking Time: 40 minutes (for cooking spaghetti squash)

Servings: 4

Ingredients:

- 1 medium-sized spaghetti squash
- 1 tablespoon olive oil
- 1 bell pepper, finely sliced
- 1 zucchini, julienned
- 1 carrot, julienned
- 1 cup cherry tomatoes, sliced
- 2 cloves garlic, minced
- 1/4 cup fresh basil, chopped
- Salt and pepper to taste
- Grated Parmesan cheese (extra, for serving)

Instructions:

- Preheat the oven to 375°F (190°C).
- After slicing the spaghetti squash in half lengthwise, remove the seeds.
- With the sliced side facing up, place the squash halves on a baking sheet. Add a drizzle of olive oil and season with pepper and salt.
- Roast the spaghetti squash in the oven for about 35-40 minutes or until the meat

easily breaks into spaghetti-like strands with a fork.

- Warm up some olive oil in a skillet over medium heat while the squash roasts. Add bell pepper, zucchini, carrot, and small tomatoes. The vegetables should be tender after 5 to 7 minutes of sautéing.
- Add the minced garlic and continue to cook for one more minute.
- Once the spaghetti squash is done, use a fork to scrape the strands into a big bowl.
- Add the sautéed veggies to the bowl with spaghetti squash. Toss everything together.
- Garnish with fresh basil and, if wanted, sliced Parmesan cheese before serving.

Nutritional Value:

(Note: Nutritional values may change based on specific products and serving sizes.)

Calories: 150 per serving, Protein: 3g, Carbohydrates: 25g, Fat: 6g, Fiber: 5g

Health Benefits:

1. As an alternative to pasta, spaghetti squash is low in calories and carbs.
2. A range of bright veggies add important nutrients and fiber.
3. Olive oil gives healthy fats.
4. Basil adds freshness and taste.

Salmon and Asparagus Foil Packets:

Preparation Time: 15 minutes.

Cooking Time: 20 minutes

Servings: 2 cups

Ingredients:

- 2 salmon chunks (6-8 oz each)
- 1 bunch asparagus, cut
- 1 lemon, finely sliced
- 2 cloves garlic, minced
- 2 cups fresh dill, chopped
- 1 tablespoon olive oil
- Salt and pepper to taste

Instructions:

- Preheat the oven to 400°F (200°C).
- Place each salmon joint in the center of a big piece of paper.
- Arrange asparagus around each salmon piece.
- Drizzle olive oil over the salmon and broccoli.
- Sprinkle sliced garlic and chopped dill over the top. Season with salt and pepper.
- Place lemon pieces on top of each salmon cut.
- Fold the foil over the fish and asparagus, making a tight box.
- Bake in the hot oven for approximately 20 minutes or until the salmon is cooked through and flakes easily.
- Carefully open the plastic bags and move the fish and broccoli to plates.

Nutritional Value:

(Note: Nutritional values may change based on specific products and serving sizes.)

Calories: 350 per serve, Protein: 30g, Carbohydrates: 10g, Fat: 20g, Fiber: 4g

Health Benefits:

1. Salmon is rich in omega-3 fatty acids, which are good for heart health.
2. Asparagus offers vitamins A, C, and K, as well as fiber.
3. Olive oil adds healthy monounsaturated fats.
4. Lemon adds a burst of lemon taste and vitamin C.

Cauliflower Fried Rice with Shrimp:

Preparation Time:15 minutes.

Cooking Time: 15 minutes

Servings: 4

Ingredients:

- 1 lb shrimp, peeled and deveined
- 1 medium-sized cauliflower, chopped or made into rice-like texture
- 1 cup frozen peas and carrots, thawed
- 2 eggs, beaten
- 3 green onions, chopped
- 3 cloves garlic, minced
- 2 tablespoons low-sodium soy sauce
- 1 tablespoon sesame oil
- 1 tablespoon olive oil
- Salt and pepper to taste

Instructions:

- In a big pan or wok, heat olive oil over medium-high heat.
- Add the shrimp, and cook for 2 to 3 minutes on each side, or until they are opaque and pink. Remove shrimp from the pan and set away. `If necessary, add a little more oil

to the same pan. Sauté garlic until fragrant.

- Add cauliflower rice to the pan and cook for 5-7 minutes, turning frequently.
- Push the cauliflower rice to the sides of the pan, forming a well in the center. Pour beaten eggs into the well and stir.
- Combine the cooked eggs with the cauliflower rice.
- Add thawed peas and carrots, cooked shrimp, and chopped green onions to the pan.
- Drizzle soy sauce and olive oil over the mixture. Stir well to blend.
- Season with salt and pepper to taste.

Nutritional Value:

(Note: Nutritional values may change based on specific products and serving sizes.)

Calories: 250 per serve, Protein: 25g, Carbohydrates: 15g, Fat: 10g, Fiber: 5g

Health Benefits:

1. Cauliflower is a low-carb option for regular rice.
2. Shrimp is a lean energy source.
3. Vegetables provide vitamins, minerals, and fiber.
4. Sesame oil adds a rich taste and healthy fats.

Black Bean and Corn Salsa Lettuce Wraps:

Preparation Time: 15 minutes.

Servings: 4

Ingredients:

- 1 can (15 oz) black beans, drained and washed
- 1 cup corn kernels (fresh, frozen, or dried)
- 1 red bell pepper, diced
- 1/2 red onion, roughly chopped
- 1 jalapeño, seeds removed and finely chopped
- 1/4 cup fresh cilantro, chopped
- Juice of 2 limes
- 1 tablespoon olive oil
- Salt and pepper to taste
- Iceberg or Romaine lettuce leaves, washed and dried

- Optional Toppings: Avocado slices, Greek yogurt or sour cream, Shredded cheese

Instructions:

- In a big bowl, mix black beans, corn, red bell pepper, red onion, jalapeño, and parsley.
- In a small bowl, mix lime juice, olive oil, salt, and pepper.
- Pour the dressing over the black bean mixture and toss well to coat.
- Spoon the black bean and corn salsa onto individual lettuce leaves, making wraps.
- Optional: Top each wrap with avocado slices, Greek yogurt or sour cream, and sliced cheese.

Nutritional Value:

(Note: Nutritional values may change based on specific products and serving sizes.)

Calories: 180 per serve, Protein: 6g , Carbohydrates: 30g, Fat: 5g, Fiber: 8g

Health Benefits:

1. Black beans are a good source of plant-based protein and fiber.
2. Corn adds natural sweetness and extra nutrients.
3. Bell peppers provide vitamin C and antioxidants.
4. Lettuce wraps lower calorie intake compared to standard wraps.

Mushroom and Spinach Stuffed Bell Peppers:

Preparation Time: 20 minutes

Cooking Time: 25 minutes

Servings: 4

Ingredients:

- 4 big bell peppers, split, and seeds removed
- 1 tablespoon olive oil
- 1 onion, roughly chopped
- 2 cloves garlic, minced
- 8 oz mushrooms, finely chopped
- 4 cups fresh spinach, chopped
- 1 cup cooked quinoa or brown rice
- 1 teaspoon dried oregano
- Salt and pepper to taste
- 1 cup tomato sauce (zero-point or low-point choice)

- 1/2 cup shredded mozzarella cheese (optional)

Instructions:

- Preheat the oven to 375°F (190°C).
- Place the bell pepper halves in a baking dish.
- In a pan, heat olive oil over medium heat. Put in the garlic and onions, and cook them until they get soft.
- Add chopped mushrooms to the pan and cook until they lose their juice.
- Stir in the chopped spinach and cook until softened.
- Remove the pan from heat and stir in cooked quinoa or brown rice, dried oregano, salt, and pepper.
- Spoon the mushroom and spinach mixture into the bell pepper halves.
- Pour tomato sauce over the stuffed peppers and, if wanted, sprinkle with shredded mozzarella cheese.
- Wrap foil around the dish and bake for 20 minutes. Remove the plastic and bake for an additional 5 minutes until the cheese is melted and bubbly.

Nutritional Value:

(Note: Nutritional values may change based on specific products and serving sizes.)

Calories: 250 per serve, Protein: 10g, Carbohydrates: 40g, Fat: 6g, Fiber: 8g

Health Benefits:

1. Bell peppers provide vitamin C and antioxidants.
2. Spinach is rich in vitamins and minerals.
3. Quinoa or brown rice adds nutrients and energy.
4. The dish is low in calories and a good source of nutrients

Lemon Garlic Shrimp Skewers:

Preparation Time:15 minutes.

Marinating Time: 30 minutes (alternative)

Cooking Time: 10 minutes

Servings: 4

Ingredients:

- 1 lb big shrimp, peeled and deveined
- Zest and juice of 2 lemons
- 3 cloves garlic, minced
- 2 tablespoons olive oil
- 1 teaspoon dried oregano
- Salt and pepper to taste
- Wooden or metal skewers
- Optional Garnish: Fresh parsley, chopped Lemon wedges

Instructions:

- If using wooden skewers, put them in water for at least 30 minutes to avoid burning.
- In a bowl, mix lemon zest, lemon juice, chopped garlic, olive oil, dried oregano, salt, and pepper to make the marinade.
- Toss the shrimp in the sauce to coat them. Allow the shrimp to marinate in the

refrigerator for 30 minutes if time allows.

- Preheat the grill or grill pan over medium-high heat.
- Thread prepared shrimp onto skewers, spreading them evenly.
- Grill the shrimp skewers for about 3-4 minutes per side or until they are dark and cooked through.
- Optional: Garnish with chopped fresh parsley and serve with lemon wedges on the side.

Nutritional Value:

(Note: Nutritional values may change based on specific products and serving sizes.)

Calories: 180 per serve, Protein: 25g, Carbohydrates: 3g, Fat: 8g, Fiber: 0g

Health Benefits:

1. Shrimp is a low-calorie and high-protein fish choice.
2. Lemon adds a pleasant lemon taste and vitamin C.
3. Garlic gives immune-boosting qualities.
4. Olive oil adds heart-healthy monounsaturated fats.

Cabbage Soup with Lean Ground Turkey:

Preparation Time: 15 minutes.

Cooking Time: 30 minutes

Servings: 6

Ingredients:

- 1 lb lean ground turkey
- 1 tablespoon olive oil

- 1 onion, diced
- 3 cloves garlic, minced
- 4 cups green cabbage, shredded
- 2 carrots, sliced
- 2 celery stalks, chopped
- 1 can (14 oz) diced tomatoes, undrained
- 6 cups low-sodium chicken or veggie soup
- 1 teaspoon dried thyme
- 1 teaspoon paprika
- Salt and pepper to taste
- Fresh parsley, chopped (for garnish)

Instructions:

- In a big pot, heat olive oil over medium heat. Add ground turkey and cook until cooked, breaking it apart with a spoon.
- Add diced onions and chopped garlic to the pot. Sauté until onions are transparent.
- Stir in shredded cabbage, sliced carrots, and chopped celery. Cook for 5 minutes until veggies start to soften.
- Pour in chopped tomatoes with their juice and add chicken or veggie broth.
- Season the soup with dried thyme, paprika, salt, and pepper. Bring to a simmer.
- Reduce heat and let the soup cook for about 20-25 minutes until the veggies are soft.
- Adjust salt to taste.
- If you want, you can add chopped fresh parsley as a garnish before serving.

Nutritional Value:

(Note: Nutritional values may change based on specific products and serving sizes.)

Calories: 200 per serve, Protein: 20g, Carbohydrates: 15g, Fat: 7g, Fiber: 5g

Health Benefits:

1. Lean ground turkey offers a good amount of energy.
2. The vitamins C and K in cabbage make it very healthy.
3. Carrots and celery add extra vitamins and minerals.
4. The soup is low in fat and calories while being full and healthy.

Egg Salad Lettuce Wraps:

Preparation Time: 15 minutes.

Servings: 4

Ingredients:

- 8 hard-boiled eggs, peeled and chopped
- 1/4 cup mayonnaise (zero-point or low-point choice)
- 1 tablespoon Dijon mustard
- 1 celery stalk, finely chopped
- 2 green onions, finely chopped
- Salt and pepper to taste
- Iceberg or Romaine lettuce leaves, washed and dried
- Optional Garnish: Paprika Fresh dill, chopped.

Instructions:

- In a big bowl, mix chopped hard-boiled eggs, mayonnaise, Dijon mustard, chopped celery, and chopped green onions.
- Mix well until all ingredients are evenly coated.

- Season with salt and pepper to taste. Adjust the mayonnaise and mustard amounts according to your taste.
- Spoon the egg salad onto individual lettuce leaves, making wraps.
- Optional: Garnish with a dash of paprika and chopped fresh dill.

Nutritional Value:

(Note: Nutritional values may change based on specific products and serving sizes.)

Calories: 200 per serve, Protein: 12g, Fat: 16g, Fiber: 1g

Health Benefits:

1. You can get a lot of good energy from eggs. Lettuce wraps lower calorie intake compared to standard wraps.
2. Celery adds crunch and is low in calories.
3. Dijon mustard offers taste without extra calories.

Caprese Stuffed Avocados:

Preparation Time: 15 minutes.

Servings: 4

Ingredients:

- 2 avocados, split and pits removed
- 1 cup cherry tomatoes, sliced
- 1 cup fresh mozzarella balls, split
- Fresh basil leaves, torn

- Balsamic glaze (zero-point or low-point choice)
- Olive oil (for dripping)
- Salt and pepper to taste
- Optional Garnish: Balsamic reduction, Freshly ground black pepper
- Instructions:
- Scoop out a little of the meat from each avocado half to make a bigger well for the stuffing.
- In a bowl, mix cherry tomatoes, fresh mozzarella, and torn basil leaves.
- Season the mixture with salt and pepper to taste. Toss gently to mix.
- Spoon the tomato and cheese mixture into the avocado halves.
- Drizzle with balsamic glaze and olive oil.
- Optional: Garnish with a vinegar sauce and freshly ground black pepper before serving.

Nutritional Value:

(Note: Nutritional values may change based on specific products and serving sizes.)

Calories: 250 per serve, Protein: 8g, Carbohydrates: 10g, Fat: 20g, Fiber: 7g

Health Benefits:

1. Avocados provide healthy natural fats and fiber.
2. Tomatoes offer vitamins C and A, as well as antioxidants.
3. Fresh mozzarella adds nutrition and a soft creaminess.
4. Basil offers a burst of taste and necessary nutrients.

<u>**Quinoa Salad with Chickpeas and Lemon-Tahini Dressing:**</u>

Preparation Time: 20 minutes

Cooking Time: 15 minutes (for rice)

Servings: 4

Ingredients

- 1 cup quinoa, rinsed
- 2 cups water or veggie soup
- 1 can (15 oz) chickpeas, drained and washed
- 1 cucumber, diced
- 1 red bell pepper, diced
- 1/2 red onion, roughly chopped
- 1/4 cup fresh parsley, chopped

For the Lemon-Tahini Dressing:

- 3 tablespoons tahini
- Juice of 2 lemons
- 2 tablespoons olive oil
- 2 cloves garlic, minced
- 1 teaspoon honey or maple syrup (optional)
- Salt and pepper to taste

Instructions:

- In a medium pot, mix rice and water or veggie broth. Bring to a boil, then reduce heat, cover, and simmer for 15 minutes or until quinoa is cooked and water is absorbed.
- In a big bowl, mix cooked rice, chickpeas, diced cucumber, diced red bell pepper, and chopped red onion.
- In a separate small bowl, mix tahini, lemon juice, olive oil, chopped garlic, honey or maple syrup (if using), salt, and pepper to make the sauce.

- After adding the dressing, thoroughly toss to coat the rice mixture.
- Garnish with chopped fresh parsley before serving.

Nutritional Value:

(Note: Nutritional values may change based on specific products and serving sizes.)

Calories: 300 per serving, Protein: 10g, Carbohydrates: 40g, Fat: 12g, Fiber: 8g

Health Benefits:

1. Quinoa is a full protein source and offers necessary amino acids.
2. Chickpeas add plant-based energy and fiber.
3. Vegetables add vitamins, minerals, and antioxidants.
4. The lemon-tahini sauce adds smoothness and good fats.

Turkey and Vegetable Stir-Fry:

Preparation Time: 15 minutes.

Cooking Time: 15 minutes

Servings: 4

Ingredients:

- 1 lb lean ground turkey
- 2 tablespoons soy sauce (low-sodium)
- 1 tablespoon oyster sauce
- 1 tablespoon hoisin sauce
- 1 tablespoon sesame oil
- 1 tablespoon vegetable oil
- 3 cups mixed veggies (broccoli sprouts, bell peppers, snap peas, carrots), chopped

- 3 cloves garlic, minced
- 1 teaspoon fresh ginger, grated
- Green onions, chopped (for garnish)
- Sesame seeds (for garnish)
- Cooked brown rice or cauliflower rice (for serving)

Instructions:

- In a small bowl, mix soy sauce, oyster sauce, and hoisin sauce. Set aside.
- In a big pan or wok, heat veggie oil and sesame oil over medium-high heat.
- Add ground turkey to the pan and cook until cooked.
- Push the turkey to one side of the pan and add garlic and ginger to the other side. Sauté until aromatic, approximately 30 seconds.
- Add mixed veggies to the pan and stir-fry for 5-7 minutes until they are crisp-tender.
- Pour the sauce over the turkey and veggies. Stir to cover everything evenly.
- Continue cooking for an additional 2-3 minutes until the sauce thickens.
- You can add chopped green onions and sesame seeds as a garnish if you want to.
- Put on top of brown rice or cauliflower rice that has been cooked.

Nutritional Value:

(Note: Nutritional values may change based on specific products and serving sizes.)

Calories: 300 per serving, Protein: 25g, Carbohydrates: 20g, Fat: 12g, Fiber: 5g

Health Benefits:

- Lean ground turkey is a high-protein, low-fat meat choice.
- Mixed veggies provide a range of vitamins and minerals.
- The stir-fry is low in calories and can be served with a healthy base like brown rice or cauliflower rice.
- Sesame oil adds a rich taste to the dish.

Sweet Potato and Black Bean Quesadillas:

Preparation Time: 20 minutes

Cooking Time: 15 minutes

Servings: 4

Ingredients:

- 2 large sweet potatoes, peeled and diced
- 1 cleaned and drained can (15 oz) of black beans
- 1 red bell pepper, diced
- 1 cup corn kernels (fresh, frozen, or dried)
- 1 teaspoon crushed cumin
- 1 teaspoon pepper spice
- Salt and pepper to taste
- 8 whole wheat or corn tortillas
- 1 cup shredded cheese (cheddar, Monterey Jack, or a mix)
- Olive oil (for food)
- Salsa, guacamole, or Greek yogurt (for serving, extra)

Instructions:

- Steam or nuke diced sweet potatoes until they are just soft.

- In a big bowl, mix steamed sweet potatoes, black beans, diced red bell pepper, and corn.
- Season the combination with ground cumin, chili powder, salt, and pepper. Toss to mix.
- Heat a pan over medium heat. Place a tortilla in the pan.
- Spread a piece of the sweet potato and black bean filling over half of the bread.
- Sprinkle shredded cheese over the center.
- Fold the bread in half, making a quesadilla. Press it down slightly with a spoon.
- Cook for 2-3 minutes on each side or until the tortilla is brown and the cheese is melted.
- Repeat the process with the leftover tortillas and filling.
- Optional: Serve with salsa, guacamole, or Greek yogurt on the side.

Nutritional Value:

(Note: Nutritional values may change based on specific products and serving sizes.)

Calories: 300 per serving, Protein: 10g, Carbohydrates: 50g, Fat: 8g, Fiber: 8g

Health Benefits:

1. Sweet potatoes provide complicated carbohydrates and are rich in vitamins.
2. Black beans add plant-based energy and nutrition.
3. Bell pepper and corn add vitamins and antioxidants.
4. Whole wheat or corn tacos offer a good form of fiber.

<u>**Chickpea and Vegetable Buddha Bowl:**</u>

Preparation Time: 20 minutes

Cooking Time: 15 minutes (for rice)

Servings: 4

Ingredients:

- 1 cup quinoa, rinsed
- 2 cups water or veggie soup
- 1 can of chickpeas, drained and rinsed
- 2 cups broccoli spears
- 2 carrots, peeled and sliced into matchsticks
- 1 red bell pepper, sliced
- 1 avocado, sliced
- 1 cucumber, sliced
- 4 cups mixed greens (spinach, kale, arugula)
- Sesame seeds (for garnish, extra)

For the Tahini Dressing:

- 1/4 cup tahini
- 2 tablespoons olive oil
- 2 tablespoons lemon juice
- 1 tablespoon maple syrup or honey
- 1 clove garlic, minced
- Salt and pepper to taste
- Water (to thin, if needed)

Instructions:

- In a medium pot, mix rice and water or veggie broth. Bring to a boil, then lower the heat, cover, and let it cook for 15 minutes, or until the water is absorbed and the quinoa is done.

- In a large pan, sauté chickpeas, broccoli, carrots, and red bell pepper over medium heat until soft veggies and chickpeas are slightly crispy.
- In a small bowl, mix tahini, olive oil, lemon juice, maple syrup or honey, chopped garlic, salt, and pepper to make the sauce. Add water as needed to achieve the required density.
- Assemble the Buddha bowls by splitting cooked quinoa, sautéed chickpeas and veggies, avocado slices, cucumber slices, and mixed greens among four bowls.
- Drizzle each bowl with tahini sauce.
- Optional: Garnish with sesame seeds.

Nutritional Value:

(Note: Nutritional values may change based on specific products and serving sizes.)

Calories: 400 per serving, Protein: 12g, Carbohydrates: 50g, Fat: 20g, Fiber: 12g

Health Benefits:

1. Quinoa is a full protein source and offers necessary amino acids.
2. Chickpeas add plant-based energy and fiber.
3. Many vitamins, minerals, and enzymes can be found in vegetables.
4. Avocado gives healthy natural fats.

Mediterranean Chickpea Salad:

Preparation Time: 15 minutes.

Servings: 4

Ingredients:

- 2 cans (15 oz each) chickpeas, drained and washed
- 1 cucumber, diced
- 1 cup cherry tomatoes, sliced
- 1/2 red onion, roughly chopped
- 1/2 cup Kalamata olives, chopped
- 1/2 cup crumbled feta cheese
- 1/4 cup fresh parsley, chopped

For the Dressing:

- 3 tablespoons extra virgin olive oil
- 2 tablespoons red wine vinegar
- 1 teaspoon dried oregano
- Salt and pepper to taste
- Lemon zest (optional)

Instructions:

- Mix beans, diced cucumber, cherry tomatoes, red onion, Kalamata olives, crumbled feta cheese, and fresh herbs in a big bowl.
- In a small bowl, mix olive oil, red wine vinegar, dried oregano, salt, and pepper to make the sauce.
- Apply the sauce to the salad and mix it gently by tossing it.
- Optional: Sprinkle lemon juice over the top before serving.

Nutritional Value:

(Note: Nutritional values may change based on specific products and serving sizes.)

Calories: 300 per serving, Protein: 12g, Carbohydrates: 30g, Fat: 15g, Fiber: 8g

Health Benefits:

1. Chickpeas provide plant-based energy and fiber.
2. Many vitamins and minerals can be found in vegetables.
3. Kalamata olives and olive oil add heart-healthy monounsaturated fats.
4. Feta cheese adds a spicy and soft flavor.

Lentil and Vegetable Soup:

Preparation Time: 15 minutes.

Cooking Time: 30 minutes

Servings: 6

Ingredients:

- **1 cup dried green or brown lentils, cleaned**
- **1 tablespoon olive oil**
- **1 onion, diced**
- **2 carrots, sliced**
- **2 celery stalks, chopped**
- **3 cloves garlic, minced**
- **1 can (14 oz) diced tomatoes, undrained**
- **6 cups vegetable broth**
- **1 teaspoon crushed cumin**
- **1 teaspoon chopped coriander**
- **1/2 teaspoon smoked pepper**
- **Salt and pepper to taste**
- **Fresh lemon pieces (for serving)**

- **Optional Garnish: Fresh parsley, chopped greek yogurt or sour cream**

Instructions:

- Bring olive oil to a medium-low temperature in a large pot. Add diced onion, sliced carrots, chopped celery, and minced garlic. Sauté until veggies are softened.
- Add washed lentils, diced tomatoes (with their juice), veggie broth, ground cumin, coriander, smoked paprika, salt, and pepper to the pot. Stir to combine.
- Bring the soup to a boil, then reduce heat and cook for 20-25 minutes or until lentils are soft.
- Adjust salt to taste.
- Optional: Garnish with chopped fresh parsley and serve with a spoonful of Greek yogurt or sour cream.
- Serve with fresh lemon wedges on the side for a burst of citrus flavor.

Nutritional Value:

(Note: Nutritional values may change based on specific products and serving sizes.)

Calories: 250 per serve, Protein: 15g, Carbohydrates: 40g, Fat: 4g, Fiber: 12g

Health Benefits:

1. Lentils provide plant-based energy and are rich in fiber.

2. A lot of different vitamins, minerals, and antioxidants can be found in vegetables.

3. Spices like cumin, coriander, and smoked paprika add taste and possible health benefits.

4. The soup is low in calories and a good source of nutrients.

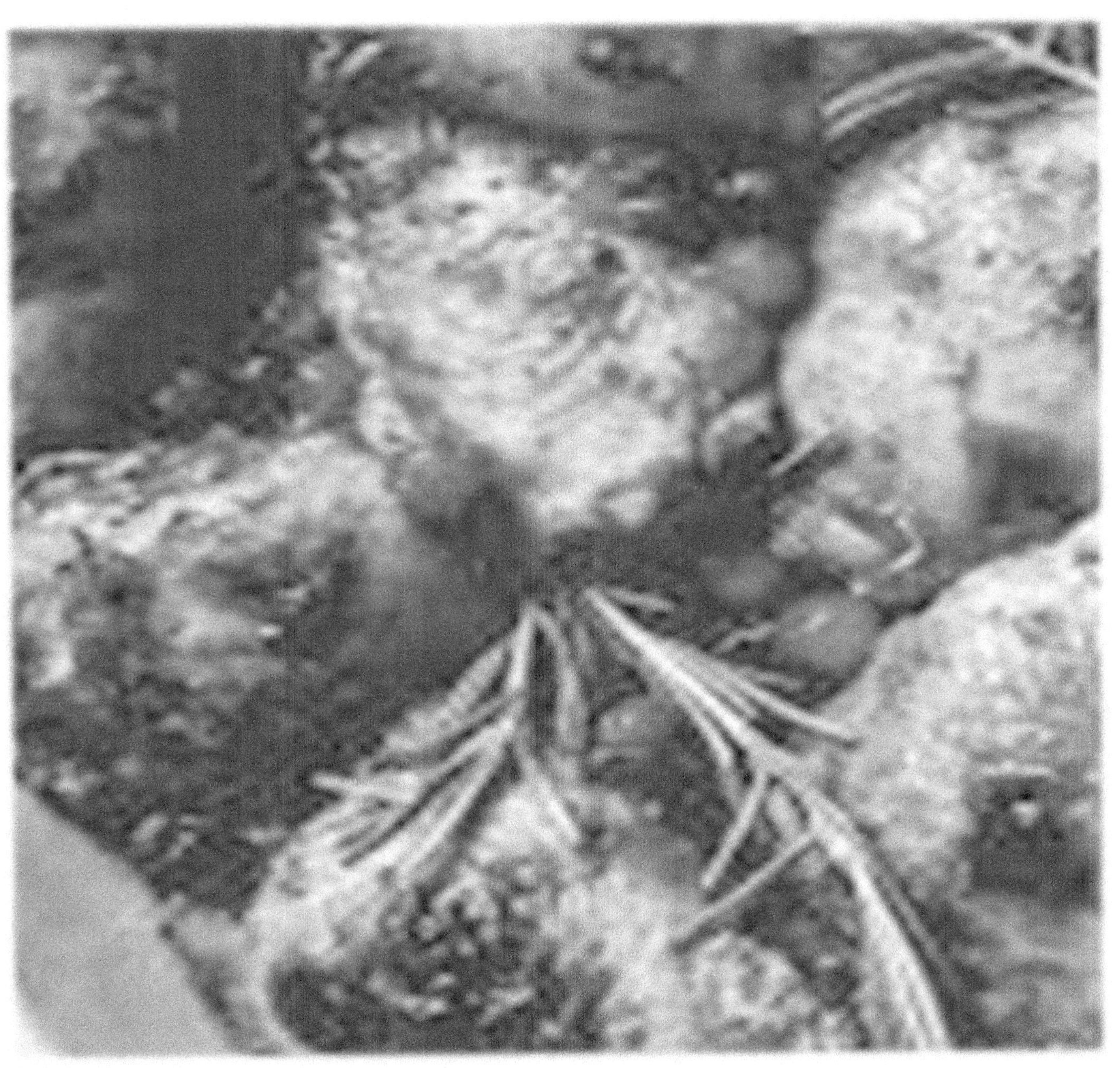

Z-P DINNER RECIPES

03

<u>**Grilled Lemon Herb Chicken:**</u>

Preparation Time: 10 minutes

Marinating Time: 30 minutes (alternative)

Cooking Time (Grilling Time): 15-20 minutes

Servings: 4

Ingredients:

- 4 boneless, skinless chicken breasts
- Zest and juice of 2 lemons
- 3 tablespoons olive oil
- 2 cloves garlic, minced
- 1 teaspoon dried thyme
- 1 teaspoon dried rosemary
- Salt and pepper to taste
- Lemon wedges (for giving)

Instructions:

- In a bowl, mix lemon zest, lemon juice, olive oil, chopped garlic, dried thyme, dried rosemary, salt, and pepper to make the marinade.
- Place chicken breasts in a sealed plastic bag or small dish and pour the marinade over them. Marinate in the refrigerator for at least 30

minutes (or longer for more taste).

- Preheat the grill to medium-high heat.
- Remove the chicken from the marinade and cook for 6-8 minutes per side or until the internal temperature hits 165°F (74°C) and the chicken is no longer pink in the center.
- Optional: Serve with lemon wedges for extra brightness.

Nutritional Value:

(Note: Nutritional values may change based on specific products and serving sizes.)

Calories: 250 per serve, Protein: 30g, Carbohydrates: 2g, Fat: 14g, Fiber: 0g

Health Benefits:

1. Chicken is a lean energy source.
2. Lemon adds a pleasant lemon taste and vitamin C.
3. Olive oil gives healthy natural fats.
4. Herbs like thyme and rosemary offer vitamins and possible health benefits.

Baked Salmon with Dill and Lemon:

Preparation Time: 10 minutes

Marinating Time: 30 minutes (alternative)

Cooking Time (Baking Time): 15-20 minutes

Servings: 4

Ingredients:

- 4 salmon pieces
- Zest and juice of 1 lemon
- 2 tablespoons olive oil
- 2 cups fresh dill, chopped
- 2 cloves garlic, minced
- Salt and pepper to taste
- Lemon slices (for topping)

Instructions:

- Preheat the oven to 400°F (200°C).
- In a bowl, mix lemon zest, lemon juice, olive oil, chopped dill, minced garlic, salt, and pepper to make the marinade.
- Place salmon pieces in a serving dish and pour the sauce over them. Marinate in the refrigerator for at least 30 minutes (or longer for more taste).
- Let the salmon come to room temperature after taking it out of the fridge.
- Bake in the prepared oven for 15-20 minutes or until the salmon flakes easily with a fork and has an internal temperature of 145°F (63°C).
- Optional: Garnish with lemon slices before serving.

Nutritional Value:

(Note: Nutritional values may change based on specific products and serving sizes.)

Calories: 300 per serving, Protein: 25g, Carbohydrates: 2g, Fat: 20g, Fiber: 0g

Health Benefits:

1. Salmon is rich in omega-3 fatty acids, which are good for heart health.
2. Lemon offers a burst of lemon taste and vitamin C.
3. Olive oil adds healthy monounsaturated fats.
4. Dill adds a fresh and flavorful part to the dish.

Vegetarian Chickpea and Spinach Curry:

Preparation Time: 15 minutcs.

Cooking Time: 20 minutes

Servings: 4

Ingredients:

- 2 tablespoons vegetable oil
- 1 onion, roughly chopped
- 3 cloves garlic, minced
- 1 tablespoon ginger, grated
- 1 can (15 oz) chickpeas, rinsed and washed
- 1 can (14 oz) diced tomatoes, undrained
- 2 tsp curry powder
- 1 teaspoon crushed cumin
- 1 teaspoon chopped coriander
- 1/2 teaspoon turmeric
- 1/2 teaspoon chili powder (change to taste)
- Salt and pepper to taste
- 1 can (14 oz) coconut milk
- 4 cups frcsh spinach, washed and chopped
- Fresh cilantro, chopped (for garnish)
- Cooked brown rice (for serving)

Instructions:

- In a big pan or pot, heat vegetable oil over medium heat. When the onion is soft, add it diced and sauté it.
- Add chopped garlic and sliced ginger to the pan. Sauté for an extra 1-2 minutes until fragrant.
- Stir in beans, diced tomatoes, curry powder, ground cumin, ground coriander, turmeric, chili powder, salt, and pepper. Cook for 5 minutes.
- Pour in coconut milk and bring the mixture to a boil. Wait 10 minutes more.
- Add chopped spinach to the pan and cook until softened.
- Adjust salt to taste.
- Optional: Serve over cooked brown rice and top with chopped fresh cilantro.

Nutritional Value:

(Note: Nutritional values may change based on specific products and serving sizes.)

Calories: 350 per serve, Protein: 10g, Carbohydrates: 30g, Fat: 20g, Fiber: 8g

Health Benefits:

1. Chickpeas provide plant-based energy and fiber.
2. Spinach is rich in vitamins and minerals.
3. Coconut milk adds smoothness and healthy fats.
4. The curry spices offer anti-inflammatory qualities.

Turkey and Quinoa Stuffed Bell Peppers:

Preparation Time: 20 minutes

Cooking Time: 30 minutes

Servings: 4

Ingredients:

- 1 cup quinoa, rinsed
- 2 cups water or veggie soup
- 1 lb lean ground turkey
- 1 tablespoon olive oil
- 1 onion, roughly chopped
- 2 cloves garlic, minced
- 1 can (14 oz) diced tomatoes, drained
- 1 cleaned and drained can (15 oz) of black beans
- 1 cup corn kernels (fresh, frozen, or dried)
- 1 teaspoon crushed cumin
- 1 teaspoon pepper spice
- Salt and pepper to taste
- 4 bell peppers, split, and seeds removed
- 1 cup shredded cheese (cheddar, Monterey Jack, or a mix)
- Fresh cilantro, chopped (for garnish)

Instructions:

- In a medium pot, mix rice and water or veggie broth. After bringing it to a boil, lower the heat, cover, and simmer the quinoa for fifteen minutes, or until it is tender and the water has been absorbed.
- In a big pan over medium heat, warm the olive oil. Add chopped onion and sliced garlic. Sauté until the onion is transparent.
- Add ground turkey to the pan and cook until browned, breaking it apart with a spoon.

- Stir in diced tomatoes, black beans, corn, ground cumin, chili powder, salt, and pepper. Cook for an extra 5 minutes.
- Preheat the oven to 375°F (190°C).
- In a mixing bowl, combine cooked rice with the turkey and veggie combination.
- Place bell pepper halves in a baking dish. Spoon the rice and turkey mixture into each pepper half.
- Top each stuffed pepper with shredded cheese.
- Bake in the hot oven for 20-25 minutes or until the peppers are soft and the cheese is melted and bubbly.
- Optional: Garnish with chopped fresh cilantro before serving.

Nutritional Value:

(Note: Nutritional values may change based on specific products and serving sizes.)

Calories: 400 per serve, Protein: 25g, Carbohydrates: 45g, Fat: 15g, Fiber: 10g

Health Benefits:

1. Quinoa offers a full source of protein and vital amino acids.
2. Lean ground turkey is a high-protein, low-fat meat choice.
3. Bell peppers offer vitamins A and C, as well as antioxidants.
4. Black beans and corn add nutrients and extra energy.

Vegetarian Zucchini Noodles with Pesto:

Preparation Time: 15 minutes.

Cooking Time: 10 minutes

Servings: 4

Ingredients:

- 4 large zucchinis, spiralized into noodles
- 2 tablespoons olive oil
- 2 cloves garlic, minced
- 1 cup cherry tomatoes, sliced
- 1/2 cup black olives, sliced
- 1/2 cup grated Parmesan cheese
- Salt and pepper to taste

For the Pesto:

- 2 cups fresh basil leaves
- 1/2 cup pine nuts, toasted
- 1/2 cup grated Parmesan cheese
- 2 cloves garlic
- 1/2 cup extra virgin olive oil
- Salt and pepper to taste
- Lemon juice (optional, for added brightness)

Instructions:

- In a food processor, mix fresh basil, toasted pine nuts, sliced Parmesan, and garlic for the pesto. Pulse until well mixed.
- With the food processor going, slowly drizzle in the olive oil until the pesto gets a smooth consistency. Season with salt and pepper to taste. Add lemon juice if necessary.
- In a big pan over medium heat, warm the olive oil. Add chopped garlic and sauté for 1-2 minutes until fragrant.
- Add zucchini noodles to the pan and toss until they are just soft, about 3-5 minutes.
- Stir in cherry tomatoes, black olives, and a large amount of

pesto. Toss until well mixed and warm through.

- Season with salt and pepper to taste.
- Serve the zucchini noodles in bowls, topped with chopped Parmesan.

Nutritional Value:

(Note: Nutritional values may change based on specific products and serving sizes.)

Calories: 250 per serve, Protein: 8g, Carbohydrates: 10g, Fat: 20g, Fiber: 5g

Health Benefits:

1. Zucchini noodles provide a low-carb option to standard pasta.
2. Pesto offers the taste of fresh basil, garlic, and pine nuts.
3. Cherry tomatoes and olives add color, vitamins, and good fats.
4. The dish is rich in healthy polyunsaturated fats and low in carbs.

Baked Chicken Parmesan:

Preparation Time: 15 minutes.

Cooking Time: 25 minutes

Servings: 4

Ingredients:

- 4 boneless, skinless chicken breasts
- Salt and pepper to taste
- 1 cup whole wheat breadcrumbs
- 1/2 cup grated Parmesan cheese

- 1 teaspoon dried oregano
- 1 teaspoon dried basil
- 1/2 teaspoon garlic powder
- 2 large eggs, beaten
- 2 cups marinara sauce (homemade or store-bought)
- 1 cup part-skim mozzarella cheese, shredded
- Fresh basil or parsley, chopped (for garnish)
- Whole wheat or multigrain spaghetti (for serving, extra)

Instructions:

- Preheat the oven to 400°F (200°C).
- Season chicken breasts with salt and pepper.
- In a small dish, mix whole wheat breadcrumbs, chopped Parmesan, dried oregano, dried basil, and garlic powder.
- Dip each chicken breast into the beaten eggs, allowing extra to drip off, then coat with the breadcrumb mixture, pressing gently to attach.
- Arrange the coated chicken onto a parchment paper-lined baking sheet.
- Bake in the hot oven for 20-25 minutes or until the chicken is cooked through and the covering is golden and crispy.
- In a small pot, heat tomato sauce over medium heat.
- Spoon a part of the tomato sauce over each chicken breast, then sprinkle with chopped cheese.
- Put the chicken back in the oven and bake it for a further five minutes, or until the cheese is bubbling and melted.

- Optional: Serve over whole wheat or multigrain spaghetti and serve with chopped fresh basil or parsley.

Nutritional Value:

(Note: Nutritional values may change based on specific products and serving sizes.)

Calories: 350 per serve: Protein: 40g; Carbohydrates: 20g, Fat: 12g, Fiber: 5g

Health Benefits:

1. Whole wheat breadcrumbs add fiber and protein.
2. Chicken is a lean source of energy.
3. Marinara sauce gives lycopene from tomatoes.
4. Mozzarella cheese adds iron and energy.

<u>Shrimp and Broccoli Stir-Fry:</u>

Preparation Time: 15 minutes.

Cooking Time: 10 minutes

Servings: 4

Ingredients:

- 1 lb big shrimp, peeled and deveined
- 2 tablespoons soy sauce (low-sodium)
- 1 tablespoon oyster sauce
- 1 tablespoon hoisin sauce
- 1 tablespoon sesame oil
- 1 tablespoon vegetable oil
- 3 cups broccoli sprouts
- 1 red bell pepper, finely sliced
- 3 cloves garlic, minced
- 1 teaspoon fresh ginger, grated

- Green onions, chopped (for garnish)
- Sesame seeds (for garnish)
- Brown rice or cauliflower rice that has been cooked (to serve)

Instructions:

- In a small bowl, mix soy sauce, oyster sauce, hoisin sauce, and olive oil. Set aside.
- In a big pan or wok, heat vegetable oil over medium-high heat.
- Add shrimp to the pan and cook for 2-3 minutes on each side until they turn pink and opaque. Remove shrimp from the pan and set away.
- If necessary, add a little more oil to the same pan. Stir in chopped garlic and grated ginger. Sauté for about 30 seconds until fragrant.
- Add broccoli sprouts and sliced red bell pepper to the pan. Stir-fry for 3-4 minutes until the veggies are crisp-tender.
- Return the cooked shrimp to the pan and pour the sauce over the mixture. Toss everything to cover evenly.
- Cook for an additional 2-3 minutes until the sauce thickens and the shrimp and veggies are well-coated.
- Optional: Garnish with chopped green onions and sesame seeds.
- Serve with cooked cauliflower rice or brown rice.

Nutritional Value:

(Note: Nutritional values may change based on specific products and serving sizes.)

Calories: 250 per serve, Protein: 25g, Carbohydrates: 15g, Fat: 10g, Fiber: 4g

Health Benefits:

1. Shrimp is a low-calorie protein source and a good source of selenium.
2. Broccoli is rich in vitamins, calcium, and antioxidants.
3. The stir-fry is low in calories and can be served with a healthy base like brown rice or cauliflower rice.
4. Sesame oil adds a rich taste to the dish.

Vegetarian Lentil and Sweet Potato Curry:

Preparation Time: 15 minutes.

Cooking Time: 25 minutes

Servings:

Ingredients:

- 1 cup dried red lentils, cleaned
- 1 big sweet potato, peeled and diced
- 1 tablespoon vegetable oil
- 1 onion, roughly chopped
- 3 cloves garlic, minced
- 1 tablespoon ginger, grated
- 2 tablespoons curry powder
- 1 teaspoon crushed cumin
- 1 teaspoon chopped coriander
- 1/2 teaspoon turmeric
- 1/2 teaspoon chili powder (change to taste)

- 1 can (14 oz) diced tomatoes, undrained
- 1 can (14 oz) coconut milk
- Salt and pepper to taste
- Fresh cilantro, chopped (for garnish)
- Cooked brown rice (for serving)

Instructions:

- In a big pot, heat vegetable oil over medium heat. When the onion is soft, add it diced and sauté it.
- Add chopped garlic and sliced ginger to the pot. Sauté for an extra 1-2 minutes until fragrant.
- Stir in curry powder, ground cumin, ground coriander, turmeric, and chili powder. Cook for 1-2 minutes to toast the spices.
- Add dried red lentils, diced sweet potato, diced tomatoes (with their juice), and coconut milk to the pot. Stir to combine.
- Bring the mixture to a simmer, then lower heat and cover. Cook for 20-25 minutes or until beans and sweet potatoes are soft.
- Season with salt and pepper to taste.
- Optional: Serve over cooked brown rice and top with chopped fresh cilantro.

Nutritional Value:

(Note: Nutritional values may change based on specific products and serving sizes.)

Calories: 350 per serve, Protein: 15g, Carbohydrates: 45g, Fat: 15g, Fiber: 10g

Health Benefits:

1. Lentils provide plant-based energy and are rich in fiber.
2. Sweet potatoes offer vitamins and complex carbs.
3. Coconut milk adds smoothness and healthy fats.
4. The curry spices offer anti-inflammatory qualities.

Beef and Vegetable Stir-Fry:

Preparation Time: 15 minutes.

Cooking Time: 15 minutes

Servings: 4

Ingredients:

- 1 lb flank steak, thinly sliced
- 3 tablespoons soy sauce (low-sodium)
- 2 tablespoons oyster sauce
- 1 tablespoon hoisin sauce
- 1 tablespoon sesame oil
- 1 tablespoon vegetable oil
- 2 bell peppers (any color), thinly sliced
- 1 big carrot, julienned
- 1 cup snap peas, cut
- 3 cloves garlic, minced
- 1 teaspoon fresh ginger, grated
- Green onions, chopped (for garnish)
- Sesame seeds (for garnish)
- Cooked brown rice or quinoa (for serving)

Instructions:

- Combine the hoisin sauce, sesame oil, oyster sauce, and soy sauce in a bowl. Set aside.
- In a big pan or wok, heat vegetable oil over medium-high heat.

- Add thinly sliced flank steak to the pan and cook for 2-3 minutes until browned. After taking the steak out of the pan, put it aside.
- If necessary, add a little more oil to the same pan. Stir in chopped garlic and grated ginger. Sauté for about 30 seconds until fragrant.
- Add bell peppers, julienned carrot, and snap peas to the pan. Stir-fry for 3-4 minutes until the veggies are crisp-tender.
- Return the cooked meat to the pan and pour the sauce over the mixture. Toss everything to cover evenly.
- Cook for an additional 2-3 minutes until the beef and veggies are well-coated and warm through.
- Optional: Garnish with chopped green onions and sesame seeds.
- Serve over cooked brown rice or quinoa.

Nutritional Value:

(Note: Nutritional values may change based on specific products and serving sizes.)

Calories: 350 per serve, Protein: 30g, Carbohydrates: 20g, Fat: 15g, Fiber: 4g

Health Benefits:

1. Flank steak is a good source of energy and iron.
2. Colorful veggies provide vitamins, minerals, and antioxidants.
3. The stir-fry is low in calories and can be made with a

healthy base like brown rice or quinoa.

4. Sesame oil adds a rich taste to the dish.

Salmon and Asparagus Foil Packets:

Preparation Time: 15 minutes

Cooking Time: 20 minutes

Servings: 4

Ingredients:

- 4 salmon pieces
- 1 lb asparagus, cut
- 2 tablespoons olive oil
- 2 cloves garlic, minced
- 1 lemon, finely sliced
- 1 teaspoon dried dill
- Salt and pepper to taste

Instructions:

- Preheat the oven to 400°F (200°C).
- Cut four big pieces of metal foil.
- In a bowl, toss cut asparagus with olive oil, crushed garlic, dried dill, salt, and pepper.
- Place a piece of asparagus in the center of each foil sheet.
- Season each salmon fillet with salt and pepper, then place a piece on top of the asparagus in each paper box.
- Top each salmon piece with a few lemon slices.
- Fold the sides of the paper over the salmon and asparagus, making a box. Seal the ends tightly.
- Place the foil bags on a baking sheet and bake in the prepared oven for 15-20 minutes or until the salmon is cooked

through and flakes easily with a fork.

- Carefully open the plastic bags, being careful of the hot steam.
- Optional: Serve with extra lemon wedges and a dash of fresh dill.

Nutritional Value:

(Note: Nutritional values may change based on specific products and serving sizes.)

Calories: 300 per serve, Protein: 25g, Carbohydrates: 10g, Fat: 18g, Fiber: 5g

Health Benefits:

1. Salmon is rich in omega-3 fatty acids, which are good for heart health.
2. Asparagus offers vitamins, minerals, and nutritional fiber.
3. Olive oil adds healthy monounsaturated fats.
4. The paper bags help seal in tastes and wetness during cooking.

Quinoa and Black Bean Stuffed Peppers:

Preparation Time: 20 minutes

Cooking Time: 30 minutes

Servings: 4

Ingredients:

- 4 big bell peppers, split and seeds removed
- 1 cup quinoa, rinsed
- 2 cups vegetable broth
- 1 tablespoon olive oil

- 1 onion, roughly chopped
- 2 cloves garlic, minced
- One can (15 oz) of rinsed and drained black beans
- 1 cup corn kernels (fresh, frozen, or dried)
- 1 teaspoon crushed cumin
- 1 teaspoon pepper spice
- 1/2 teaspoon smoked pepper
- Salt and pepper to taste
- 1 cup salsa
- 1 cup shredded cheese (cheddar, Monterey Jack, or a mix)
- Fresh cilantro, chopped (for garnish)

Instructions:

- Preheat the oven to 375°F (190°C).
- Place split bell peppers in a baking dish.
- In a medium pot, mix rice and veggie broth. After bringing to a boil, lower the heat, cover the pot, and simmer the quinoa for fifteen minutes, or until the liquid has been absorbed.
- Over medium heat, warm the olive oil in a big pan. When the onion is soft, add it diced and sauté it.
- Add chopped garlic to the pan and sauté for an additional 1-2 minutes until fragrant.
- Stir in black beans, corn, ground cumin, chili powder, smoked paprika, salt, and pepper. Cook for 5 minutes.
- Combine the cooked rice with the black bean sauce in the pan. Mix well.

- Spoon the rice and black bean mixture into each bell pepper half.
- Top each stuffed pepper with salsa and chopped cheese.
- Bake in the hot oven for 20-25 minutes or until the peppers are soft and the cheese is melted and bubbly.
- Optional: Garnish with chopped fresh cilantro before serving.

Nutritional Value:

(Note: Nutritional values may change based on specific products and serving sizes.)

Calories: 350 per serve, Protein: 15g, Carbohydrates: 55g, Fat: 10g, Fiber: 12g

Health Benefits:

1. Quinoa offers a full source of protein and vital amino acids.
2. Black beans add protein, fiber, and important nutrients.
3. Bell peppers offer vitamins A and C, as well as antioxidants.
4. The dish is high in fiber and low in heavy fats.

Mushroom and Spinach Stuffed Chicken Breast:

Preparation Time: 20 minutes

Cooking Time: 25 minutes

Servings: 4

Ingredients:

- 4 boneless, skinless chicken breasts
- Salt and pepper to taste
- 1 tablespoon olive oil

- 2 cups mushrooms, finely chopped
- 2 cups fresh spinach, chopped
- 2 cloves garlic, minced
- 1/2 cup feta cheese, chopped
- 1/4 cup Parmesan cheese, grated
- 1 teaspoon dried thyme
- 1 teaspoon dried rosemary
- 1/2 cup low-sodium chicken soup
- Lemon wedges (for giving)

Instructions:

- Preheat the oven to 400°F (200°C).
- Season chicken breasts with salt and pepper.
- In a big pan over medium heat, warm the olive oil. Once the onion is tender, chop it and sauté it.
- Add chopped mushrooms to the pan and sauté until they lose their wetness and become golden brown.
- Stir in minced garlic and chopped spinach. Cook for 2-3 minutes until spinach is wilted.
- Remove the pan from heat and let the mushroom and spinach mixture cool slightly.
- Add feta cheese, Parmesan cheese, dried thyme, and dried rosemary to the mixture. Mix well.
- Cut a hole into each chicken breast by slicing horizontally, being careful not to cut all the way through.
- Stuff each chicken breast with the mushroom and spinach filling.

- Secure the holes with toothpicks or kitchen twine.
- Return the pan to medium-high heat. Brown the stuffed chicken breasts for 2-3 minutes on each side.
- Pour chicken stock into the pan and move it to the prepared oven.
- Bake for 20-25 minutes or until the chicken is cooked through and gets an internal temperature of 165°F (74°C).
- Optional: Serve with lemon wedges for a burst of citrus taste.

Nutritional Value:

(Note: Nutritional values may change based on specific products and serving sizes.)

Calories: 300 per serving, Protein: 35g, Carbohydrates: 5g, Fat: 15g, Fiber: 2g

Health Benefits:

1. Chicken breast is a lean source of energy.
2. Mushrooms and spinach provide vitamins, minerals, and antioxidants.
3. Feta and Parmesan cheese add a rich taste and protein.
4. The dish is low in sugar and a good source of important nutrients.

Eggplant Parmesan:

Preparation Time: 30 minutes

Cooking Time: 40 minutes

Servings: 4

Ingredients:

- 2 large eggplants, sliced into 1/2-inch rounds
- Salt for drying the eggplant
- 2 cups marinara sauce (homemade or store-bought)
- 1 cup part-skim mozzarella cheese, shredded
- 1/2 cup Parmesan cheese, grated
- 1 cup whole wheat breadcrumbs
- 2 teaspoons dried oregano
- 1 teaspoon dried basil
- 1/2 teaspoon garlic powder
- Olive oil spray
- Fresh basil, chopped (for garnish)
- Whole wheat noodles (for serving, extra)

Instructions:

- Preheat the oven to 375°F (190°C).
- Place eggplant slices on a baking sheet and sprinkle each slice with salt. Let them sit for 15-20 minutes to release extra liquid.
- Pat the eggplant slices dry with a paper towel to remove the released wetness.
- In a bowl, mix whole wheat breadcrumbs, dried oregano, dried basil, and garlic powder.
- Dip each eggplant slice into the breadcrumb mixture, pressing gently to attach.
- Arrange the fried eggplant slices onto a parchment paper-lined baking sheet.
- Spray the top of each slice with olive oil spray.

- Bake in the hot oven for 25-30 minutes or until the eggplant is golden and crispy.
- In a serving dish, spread a thin layer of tomato sauce.
- Spread some roasted eggplant slices over the sauce.
- Sprinkle with a piece of shredded mozzarella and chopped Parmesan.
- Repeat the steps, ending with a layer of cheese on top.
- Bake for an extra 15-20 minutes or until the cheese is melted and bubbly.
- Optional: Serve over whole wheat spaghetti and top with chopped fresh basil.

Nutritional Value:

(Note: Nutritional values may change based on specific products and serving sizes.)

Calories: 300 per serving, Protein: 15g, Carbohydrates: 30g, Fat: 12g, Fiber: 8g

Health Benefits:

1. Eggplant is a low-calorie veggie rich in fiber.
2. Whole wheat breadcrumbs add fiber and protein.
3. Marinara sauce gives lycopene from tomatoes.
4. Mozzarella and Parmesan cheese add iron and protein.

Lemon Garlic Shrimp Pasta:

Preparation Time: 15 minutes.

Cooking Time: 15 minutes

Servings: 4

Ingredients:

- 8 oz whole wheat or multigrain spaghetti
- 1 lb big shrimp, peeled and deveined
- Salt and pepper to taste
- 3 tablespoons olive oil
- 4 cloves garlic, minced
- One teaspoon of red pepper flakes, optional for further spiciness
- Zest of 1 lemon
- Juice of 1 lemon
- 1/2 cup cherry tomatoes, split
- 1/4 cup fresh parsley, chopped
- Grated Parmesan cheese (for dish)

Instructions:

- Cook the whole wheat or multigrain spaghetti according to package directions. Drain and set away.
- Season shrimp with salt and pepper.
- In a big pan, warm the olive oil over medium-high heat.
- Add shrimp to the pan and cook for 2-3 minutes on each side until they turn pink and opaque. Remove shrimp from the pan and set away.
- Add a little more oil to the same pan if necessary. Add chopped garlic and red pepper flakes (if using). Sauté for about 30 seconds until fragrant.
- Stir in lemon peel and lemon juice. Cook for an extra 1-2 minutes.
- Add cooked spaghetti to the pan and toss to coat with the lemon-garlic sauce.

- Stir in cherry tomatoes and cooked shrimp. Toss until well mixed and warm through.
- Season with extra salt and pepper to taste.
- Sprinkle chopped fresh parsley over the pasta.
- Optional: Serve with chopped Parmesan cheese.

Nutritional Value:

(Note: Nutritional values may change based on specific products and serving sizes.)

Calories: 350 per serve, Protein: 25g, Carbohydrates: 40g, Fat: 12g, Fiber: 8g

Health Benefits:

1. Whole wheat or multigrain pasta adds fiber and calories.
2. Shrimp is a low-calorie protein source and a good source of selenium.
3. Lemon offers a burst of lemon taste and vitamin C.
4. Fresh herbs like parsley add vitamins and antioxidants.

Turkey and Vegetable Chili:

Preparation Time: 20 minutes

Cooking Time: 30 minutes

Servings: 6

Ingredients:

- 1 lb lean ground turkey
- 1 tablespoon olive oil
- 1 onion, chopped

- 2 bell peppers (any color), chopped
- 2 carrots, peeled and diced
- 3 cloves garlic, minced
- One can (15 oz) of rinsed and drained black beans
- 1 can (15 oz) kidney beans, drained and washed
- 1 can (14 oz) diced tomatoes, undrained
- 1 cup corn kernels (fresh, frozen, or dried)
- 2 tablespoons tomato sauce
- 1 cup low-sodium chicken or veggie soup
- 2 tablespoons pepper spice
- 1 teaspoon crushed cumin
- 1 teaspoon dried oregano
- 1/2 teaspoon smoked pepper
- Salt and pepper to taste
- Fresh cilantro, chopped (for garnish)
- Greek yogurt or low-fat sour cream (for serving)

Instructions:

- Olive oil should be heated on medium heat in a large saucepan. Add chopped onion, bell peppers, and carrots. Sauté until veggies are softened.
- Add chopped garlic to the pot and sauté for an additional 1-2 minutes until fragrant.
- Break up the ground turkey with a spoon while you cook it until it becomes brown.
- Stir in chili powder, ground cumin, dried oregano, smoked paprika, salt, and pepper. Cook for 1-2 minutes to toast the spices.
- Toss in the tomato paste and stir well.

- Pour in chopped tomatoes, black beans, kidney beans, corn, and chicken or veggie broth. Stir to combine.
- Bring the chili to a simmer, then reduce heat and cover. Let it boil for 20-25 minutes to allow the spices to mix and the chili to thicken.
- Season with extra salt and pepper to taste.
- Optional: Garnish with chopped fresh cilantro before serving.
- Serve the chili hot, with a spoonful of Greek yogurt or low-fat sour cream if preferred.

Nutritional Value:

(Note: Nutritional values may change based on specific products and serving sizes.)\

Calories: 300 per serving, Protein: 25g, Carbohydrates: 30g, Fat: 10g, Fiber: 8g

Health Benefits:

1. Lean ground turkey is a high-protein, low-fat meat choice.
2. Beans add bulk and extra energy.
3. Vegetables provide vitamins, minerals, and antioxidants.
4. The soup is a filling and satisfying choice for a healthy dinner.

Sweet Potato and Chickpea Curry:

Preparation Time: 20 minutes

Cooking Time: 30 minutes

Servings: 4

Ingredients:

- 2 large sweet potatoes, peeled and diced
- One can (15 oz) rinsed, drained, and mashed chickpeas
- 1 tablespoon vegetable oil
- 1 onion, roughly chopped
- 3 cloves garlic, minced
- 1 tablespoon fresh ginger, chopped
- 2 tablespoons curry powder
- 1 teaspoon crushed cumin
- 1 teaspoon chopped coriander
- 1/2 teaspoon turmeric
- 1/2 teaspoon chili pepper (change to taste)
- 1 can (14 oz) diced tomatoes, undrained
- 1 can (14 oz) coconut milk
- Salt and pepper to taste
- Fresh cilantro, chopped (for garnish)
- Cooked brown rice (for serving)

Instructions:

- In a big pot, heat vegetable oil over medium heat. Add chopped onion and cook until it becomes tender.
- Add chopped garlic and sliced ginger to the pot. Sauté for an extra 1-2 minutes until fragrant.
- Stir in curry powder, ground cumin, ground coriander, turmeric, and chili pepper. Cook for 1-2 minutes to toast the spices.
- Add diced sweet potatoes, chickpeas, chopped tomatoes (with their juice), and coconut

milk to the pot. Stir to combine.

- Bring the mixture to a simmer, then lower the heat and cover. Cook sweet potatoes for 20 to 25 minutes, or until they are tender.
- Season with salt and pepper to taste.
- Optional: Serve over cooked brown rice and top with chopped fresh cilantro.

Nutritional Value:

(Note: Nutritional values may change based on specific products and serving sizes.)

Calories: 350 per serve, Protein: 10g, Carbohydrates: 45g, Fat: 15g, Fiber: 8g

Health Benefits:

1. Sweet potatoes provide vitamins, minerals, and complicated carbs.
2. Chickpeas add plant-based energy and fiber.
3. Coconut milk adds smoothness and healthy fats.
4. The curry spices offer anti-inflammatory qualities.

Mediterranean Quinoa Salad:

Preparation Time: 20 minutes

Cooking Time: 15 minutes (for rice)

Servings: 4

Ingredients:

- 1 cup quinoa, rinsed
- 2 cups water or veggie soup
- 1 cup cherry tomatoes, sliced

- 1 cucumber, diced
- 1/2 cup Kalamata olives, chopped
- 1/2 cup red onion, finely chopped
- 1/2 cup crumbled feta cheese
- 1/4 cup fresh parsley, chopped
- 1/4 cup fresh mint, chopped
- 3 tablespoons extra-virgin olive oil
- 2 tablespoons red wine vinegar
- 1 teaspoon dried oregano
- Salt and pepper to taste
- Lemon wedges (for giving)

Instructions:

- Rinse quinoa under cold water. In a pot, mix rice and water or veggie broth. After bringing to a boil, lower the heat, cover the pot, and simmer the quinoa for fifteen minutes, or until the liquid has been absorbed. Using a fork, fluff and let to cool.
- In a big bowl, mix cooked quinoa, cherry tomatoes, cucumber, Kalamata olives, red onion, feta cheese, fresh parsley, and fresh mint.
- In a small bowl, mix together extra-virgin olive oil, red wine vinegar, dried oregano, salt, and pepper to make the sauce.
- Pour the dressing over the rice mixture and toss to coat everything evenly.
- Season with extra salt and pepper to taste.
- Serving lemon wedges on the side is optional.

Nutritional Value:

(Note: Nutritional values may change based on specific products and serving sizes.)

Calories: 350 per serve, Protein: 10g, Carbohydrates: 35g, Fat: 20g, Fiber: 5g

Health Benefits

1. Quinoa offers a full source of protein and vital amino acids.
2. Mediterranean foods offer a range of vitamins, minerals, and antioxidants.
3. Olive oil adds healthy monounsaturated fats.
4. Feta cheese offers protein and a rich taste.

Chicken and Vegetable Stir-Fry with Cashews:

Preparation Time: 20 minutes

Cooking Time: 15 minutes

Servings: 4

Ingredients:

- One pound of finely sliced, boneless, skinless chicken breasts
- Salt and pepper to taste
- 2 tablespoons soy sauce (low-sodium)
- 1 tablespoon oyster sauce
- 1 tablespoon hoisin sauce
- 1 tablespoon cornstarch
- 2 tablespoons vegetable oil, split
- 1 bell pepper, finely sliced (any color)
- 1 zucchini, chopped
- 1 cup broccoli stems
- 1 cup snap peas, cut
- 3 cloves garlic, minced
- 1 teaspoon fresh ginger, grated
- 1/2 cup raw cashews

- Green onions, chopped (for garnish)
- Cooked brown rice or quinoa (for serving)

Instructions:

- Season chicken pieces with salt and pepper.
- In a bowl, mix together soy sauce, oyster sauce, hoisin sauce, and cornstarch to make the sauce. Set aside.
- Heat 1 tablespoon of vegetable oil in a wok or big pan over high heat.
- Add chicken slices to the hot wok and stir-fry for 3-4 minutes until browned and cooked through. Remove the chicken and transfer it to a platter.
- In the same pan, add another tablespoon of oil if needed.
- Add chopped garlic and grated ginger. Sauté for about 30 seconds until fragrant.
- Add bell pepper, zucchini, broccoli pieces, and snap peas to the wok. Stir-fry for 3-4 minutes until the veggies are crisp-tender.
- Return the cooked chicken to the wok and pour the sauce over the mixture. Toss everything to cover evenly.
- Add raw peanuts to the wok and stir to mix.
- Cook for an additional 2-3 minutes until the chicken and veggies are well-coated and warm through.
- Optional: Garnish with chopped green onions.
- Serve over cooked brown rice or quinoa.

Nutritional Value:

(Note: Nutritional values may change based on specific products and serving sizes.)

Calories: 400 per serve, Protein: 30g, Carbohydrates: 30g, Fat: 18g, Fiber: 5g

Health Benefits:

1. Chicken breast is a lean source of energy.
2. Cashews provide healthy fats and a delicious taste.
3. Colorful veggies offer vitamins, minerals, and antioxidants.
4. The stir-fry is low in calories and can be made with a healthy base like brown rice or quinoa.

Vegetarian Lentil and Spinach Stuffed Bell Peppers:

Preparation Time: 20 minutes

Cooking Time: 30 minutes

Servings: 4

Ingredients:

- 1 cup dry green or brown lentils, cleaned
- 2 1/2 cups veggie broth
- 4 big bell peppers, split and seeds removed
- 1 tablespoon olive oil
- 1 onion, roughly chopped
- 2 cloves garlic, minced
- 1 can (14 oz) diced tomatoes, drained
- 2 cups fresh spinach, chopped
- 1 teaspoon crushed cumin
- 1 teaspoon smoked pepper
- Salt and pepper to taste

- 1 cup shredded mozzarella cheese
- Fresh parsley, chopped (for garnish)
- Cooked quinoa or brown rice (for serving)

Instructions:

- In a pot, mix beans and veggie broth. Bring to a boil, then reduce heat, cover, and cook for 20-25 minutes or until lentils are soft. Drain any extra liquid.
- Preheat the oven to 375°F (190°C).
- Place split bell peppers in a baking dish.
- Olive oil should be heated at medium heat in a large pan. When the onion is soft, add it diced and sauté it.
- Add chopped garlic to the pan and sauté for an additional 1-2 minutes until fragrant.
- Stir in diced tomatoes, chopped spinach, ground cumin, smoked paprika, salt, and pepper. Cook for 3-4 minutes until the spinach is soft.
- Add cooked beans to the pan and mix well.
- Spoon the bean and spinach mixture into each bell pepper half.
- Place shredded mozzarella cheese on top of each filled pepper.
- Bake in the hot oven for 20-25 minutes or until the peppers are soft and the cheese is melted and bubbly.

- Optional: Before serving, sprinkle some freshly chopped parsley on top.
- Serve over cooked quinoa or brown rice.

Nutritional Value:

(Note: Nutritional values may change based on specific products and serving sizes.)

Calories: 350 per serve, Protein: 20g, Carbohydrates: 50g, Fat: 10g, Fiber: 15g

Health Benefits:

1. Lentils provide plant-based energy and are rich in fiber.
2. Bell peppers offer vitamins A and C, as well as antioxidants.
3. Spinach adds iron, vitamins, and minerals.

4. The dish is a healthy and filling meatless choice.

Grilled Lemon Herb Chicken with Quinoa Salad:

Preparation Time: 15 minutes.

Marinating Time: 30 minutes

Cooking Time: 15 minutes

Servings: 4

Ingredients:

For Grilled Lemon Herb Chicken:

- 4 boneless, skinless chicken breasts
- Zest and juice of 2 lemons
- 3 tablespoons olive oil
- 2 cloves garlic, minced

- 1 teaspoon dried oregano
- 1 teaspoon dried thyme
- Salt and pepper to taste

For Quinoa Salad:

- 1 cup quinoa, rinsed
- 2 cups water or veggie soup
- 1 cucumber, diced
- 1 pint cherry tomatoes, split
- 1/2 red onion, roughly chopped
- 1/4 cup fresh parsley, chopped
- 1/4 cup fresh mint, chopped
- dried thyme, salt, and pepper to make the marinate.
- Place chicken breasts in a small dish and pour half of the marinate over them. Let it marinate for a minimum of half an hour in the fridge.
- Turn the heat up to medium-high on the grill or grill pan.

- 3 tablespoons extra-virgin olive oil
- 2 tablespoons red wine vinegar
- Salt and pepper to taste

Instructions:

For Grilled Lemon Herb Chicken:

- In a bowl, mix together lemon zest, lemon juice, olive oil, chopped garlic, dried oregano,

- Grill the chicken breasts for 6-7 minutes on each side or until fully cooked and grill marks show. Discard the used sauce.
- Optional: Baste the chicken with the leftover sauce during cooking.

For Quinoa Salad:

- In a pot, mix rice and water or veggie broth. After bringing to a boil, lower the heat, cover the pot, and simmer the quinoa for fifteen minutes, or until the liquid has been absorbed. Using a fork, fluff and let to cool.

- In a big bowl, mix cooked quinoa, diced cucumber, cherry tomatoes, chopped red onion, fresh parsley, and fresh mint.
- In a small bowl, mix together extra-virgin olive oil, red wine vinegar, salt, and pepper to make the sauce.
- Pour the dressing over the quinoa salad and toss to coat everything evenly.
- Season with extra salt and pepper to taste.

Nutritional Value:

(Note: Nutritional values may change based on specific products and serving sizes.)

Calories: 400 per serve, Protein: 30g, Carbohydrates: 30g, Fat: 18g, Fiber: 5g

Health Benefits:

1. Chicken breast is a lean source of energy.
2. Quinoa adds protein and vital amino acids.
3. Vegetables in the salad provide vitamins, minerals, and antioxidants.
4. Olive oil in the sauce adds healthy monounsaturated fats.

04

Stuffed Bell Peppers with Quinoa

Preparation Time: 20 minutes

Cooking Time: 40 minutes

Servings: 4.

Ingredients:

- Four bell peppers, any hue
- One cup of cooked quinoa
- chopped veggies, including zucchini, onions, and carrots
- mildly salted tomato sauce
- fresh herbs, like basil or parsley
- To taste, add salt and pepper.
- Vegan cheese is optional (for topping)

Instructions:

- Turn the oven on to 375°F, or 190°C.
- Slice off the bell peppers' tops, then take out the seeds and membranes.
- Combine cooked quinoa, tomato sauce, chopped

veggies, fresh herbs, and seasonings in a bowl.

- Stuff the quinoa mixture inside each bell pepper.
- The filled peppers should be put on a roasting tray. For 30 to 35 minutes, bake with a foil cover on.
- Take off the foil, cover with the vegan cheese of your choice, and bake for a further five minutes, or until the cheese has melted.

Pesto with Zucchini Noodles

Preparation Time: 15 minutes.

Cooking Time: 5 minutes

Servings: 2.

Ingredients:

Nutritional Value (Per Serving):

Approximately 150 calories, 5g of protein, 30g of carbohydrates, Fat: 1 gram, 7g of fiber

Health Benefits:

1. High in Fiber and Protein: Quinoa helps with digestion and fullness by providing both fiber and protein.

Bell peppers are low in calories but high in vital vitamins and minerals. They are also rich in nutrients.

- two medium-sized zucchini
- homemade or low-fat pesto sauce from the supermarket
- Half a cherry tomato
- (Optional) pine nuts
- For garnish, use fresh basil leaves.
- To taste, add salt and pepper.

- Instructions:

- To make zucchini noodles, use a vegetable peeler or spiralizer.
- The zucchini noodles should be softened somewhat after three to five minutes of gentle sautéing in a skillet over medium heat.
- Once the zucchini noodles are properly coated, toss them in the pesto sauce.
- Add the cherry tomatoes and, if using, the pine nuts. Gently mix everything together.
- Add pepper and salt for seasoning.
- Before serving, garnish with fresh basil leaves.

Nutritional Value (Per Serving)::

Approximately 120 calories, 3g of protein, 10g of carbohydrates, 8g of fat, 3g of fiber

Health Benefits:

1) Low-Calorie Substitute: Instead of regular spaghetti, zucchini noodles are a low-calorie option.
2) Rich in Vitamins: Zucchinis provide a nutrient-dense diet since they are high in vitamins and minerals.

Salad with Black Beans and Corn

Preparation Time: 15 minutes.

4-6 servings in total

Ingredients:

- Black beans, washed and drained, in one can (15 ounces).
- One cup of fresh or, if frozen, thawed corn kernels

- One sliced red bell pepper
- Half a red onion, cut finely
- Diced and seeded jalapeño (optional for heat)
- chopped fresh cilantro
- two limes' worth of juice
- Two tsp olive oil
- To taste, add salt and pepper.
- Avocado: a garnish that is optional

Instructions:

- Black beans, corn, diced red bell pepper, sliced red onion, diced jalapeño (if used), and fresh cilantro should all be combined in a large mixing dish.
- Mix the lime juice, olive oil, salt, and pepper in a separate small bowl.
- After pouring the dressing over the bean mixture, toss to fully incorporate.
- If necessary, taste and adjust the seasoning.
- If desired, garnish with sliced avocado just before serving.

Nutritional Value (Per Serving):

Approximately 150 calories, 6g of protein, 23g of carbohydrates, 5g of fat, 6g of fiber

Health Benefits:

1. Rich in Protein and Fiber: Black beans are a great source of both protein and fiber.
2. Vitamin-Packed: This salad promotes general health since it is full of vitamins from a variety of veggies.

Fried rice with cauliflower

Preparation Time: 15 minutes.

Cooking Time: 10 minutes

Servings: 4.

Ingredients:

- One medium head of cauliflower, finely chopped or processed until it resembles rice.
- One cup of mixed veggies (corn, carrots, and peas)
- two minced garlic cloves
- One little onion, diced finely
- Two teaspoons of tamari or low-sodium soy sauce
- One tablespoon of sesame oil
- Two sliced green onions (for garnish)
- Optional sesame seeds for garnish
- To taste, add salt and pepper.

Instructions:

- Heat the sesame oil in a big skillet or wok over medium heat.
- Add the chopped onion and minced garlic, and sauté until the onions become transparent and aromatic.
- When the mixed veggies begin to soften, add them and continue to simmer.
- When the cauliflower rice achieves the appropriate softness, stir-fry it for five to seven minutes after adding it.
- Stirring to ensure smooth blending, drizzle soy sauce over the mixture. Add pepper and salt for seasoning.
- Before serving, garnish with sesame seeds and finely chopped green onions.

Nutritional Value (Per Serving):

Approximately 100 calories, 5g of protein, 15g of carbohydrates, 3g of fat, 5g of fiber

Health Benefits:

1. Low-Carb Substitute: An alternative to regular rice that is low in carbohydrates is cauliflower rice.
2. Rich in Vitamins: This meal is full of veggies that provide a range of vitamins and minerals.

Curry with Chickpeas and Spinach

Preparation Time: 10 minutes

Cooking Time: 20 minutes

Servings: 4.

Ingredients:

- Two cans of washed and drained chickpeas, 15 ounces each
- One onion, chopped finely
- three minced garlic cloves
- one tsp finely chopped ginger
- One can of chopped tomatoes (14 ounces)
- Two cups of raw spinach
- One 14-ounce can of coconut milk
- Curry powder, two teaspoons
- one tsp finely ground turmeric
- One teaspoon of cumin powder
- One tablespoon of olive oil
- To taste, add salt and pepper.
- To garnish, use fresh cilantro.

Instructions:

- In a big pan, warm up the olive oil over medium heat. Sauté the chopped onion until it becomes transparent.

- Add the grated ginger and minced garlic, and simmer for an additional minute, or until fragrant.
- Add the ground cumin, turmeric, and curry powder and stir. Cook for one to two minutes.
- Add the coconut milk, chickpeas, and chopped tomatoes. Simmer for ten minutes.
- After adding the fresh spinach, simmer it for a further five minutes, or until it wilts.
- Season with salt and pepper, to taste.
- Before serving, garnish with fresh cilantro.

Nutritional Value (Per Serving):

Approximately 160 calories, 6g of protein, 18g of carbohydrates, 8g of fat, 6g of fiber

Health Benefits:

1. Rich in Protein and Fiber: The protein and fiber included in chickpeas help with digestion and satiety.
2. Vitamin-Packed: A nutrient-dense meal is enhanced by the abundance of vitamins and minerals found in spinach.

Portobello Mushrooms Stuffed

Preparation Time: 15 minutes.

Cooking Time: 20 minutes

Servings: 4.

Ingredients:

- Removed stems from four huge Portobello mushrooms.

- One cup of finely chopped spinach
- half a cup of chopped cherry tomatoes
- diced red bell pepper, half a cup
- 1/4 cup of coarsely chopped red onion
- two minced garlic cloves
- Half a cup of whole wheat breadcrumbs (for a healthy choice)
- 1/4 cup grated Parmesan cheese (may be substituted with vegan cheese if desired)
- Two tsp olive oil
- For garnish, use fresh basil leaves.
- To taste, add salt and pepper.

Instructions:

- Turn the oven on to 375°F, or 190°C. The Portobello mushrooms should be put on a baking pan.
- With a pan over medium heat, preheat the olive oil. Add the minced garlic and sauté it until fragrant.
- Add the cherry tomatoes, red onion, red bell pepper, and chopped spinach. Simmer the veggies for 3 to 4 minutes, or until they are tender. Add the breadcrumbs and, if using, the grated Parmesan cheese. Simmer for one more minute.
- Stuff the veggie mixture into each cap of a Portobello mushroom.
- Bake for 15 to 20 minutes, or until the filling is golden brown and the mushrooms are soft.
- Before serving, garnish with fresh basil leaves.

Nutritional Value (Per Serving):

Approximately 130 calories, 5g of protein, 14g of carbohydrates, 7g of fat, 4g of fiber

Health Benefits:

1. Portobello mushrooms are rich in fiber and low in calories, which helps with digestion.
2. Rich in Nutrients: This meal is loaded with a variety of veggies that provide vital vitamins and minerals.

Tomato and Eggplant Bake

Preparation Time: 20 minutes

Cooking Time: 30 minutes

Servings: 4.

Ingredients:

- Cut two medium eggplants into rounds.
- Four sliced tomatoes
- two minced garlic cloves
- 1/4 cup finely chopped fresh basil leaves
- 1/4 cup finely chopped fresh parsley
- 1/4 cup grated Parmesan cheese (may be substituted with vegan cheese if desired)
- Two tsp olive oil
- To taste, add salt and pepper.

Instructions:

- Turn the oven on to 375°F, or 190°C. Spread some olive oil on a baking dish.
- Arrange the rounds of eggplant in a layer at the base of the baking dish.

- Add chopped garlic, sliced tomatoes, parsley, and fresh basil to the eggplant's surface.
- Add a drizzle of olive oil and season with pepper and salt.
- Bake the dish for 20 minutes with the foil covering it.
- When the eggplant is soft and the cheese is golden, remove the cover, scatter over the grated Parmesan cheese, if using, and bake for a further ten minutes.

Nutritional Value (Per Serving):

Approximately 120 calories, 4g of protein, 16g of carbohydrates, 6g of fat, 8g of fiber

Health Benefits:

1. Low in calories and high in nutrients: Eggplants are a good source of fiber and antioxidants, two important nutrients.

2. Tomatoes are a vegetable that is high in vitamins, particularly vitamin C, which is good for your general health.

Stir-fried vegetables with tofu

Preparation Time: 15 minutes .

Cooking Time: 15 minutes

Servings: 4.

Ingredients:

- One block of diced and pressed firm tofu
- Two cups of mixed veggies, including carrots, snap peas, broccoli, and bell peppers
- One sliced onion
- three minced garlic cloves
- One tablespoon of grated ginger
- Three tablespoons of tamari or low-sodium soy sauce
- One-tspn rice vinegar

- One tablespoon of sesame oil
- 1 tablespoon cornstarch (two tablespoons water combined)
- Garnish with 2 tablespoons of finely chopped green onions
- Add a garnish of sesame seeds (optional).
- To taste, add salt and pepper.

Instructions:

- In a large skillet or wok, heat the sesame oil over medium-high heat.
- Stir-fry the cubed tofu until it becomes golden brown on both sides. Take out the tofu and put it aside.
- Add the minced garlic, grated ginger, and sliced onion to the same pan. Sauté until aromatic, about 1 minute.
- When the mixed veggies begin to soften, add them to the skillet and stir-fry for three to four minutes.
- Combine the cornstarch-water combination, rice vinegar, and soy sauce in a small bowl. Drizzle the veggies with it.
- Reintroduce the cooked tofu to the pan and stir everything until the sauce is thicker.
- Season with salt and pepper, to taste.
- Before serving, garnish with sesame seeds and finely chopped green onions.

Nutritional Value (Per Serving):

Approximately 150 calories, 10g of protein, 12g of carbohydrates, 8g of fat, 4g of fiber

Health and Nutritional benefits:

1. High-Protein: Tofu is an excellent plant-based protein source.
2. Vitamin-Rich: The nutritional profile is improved by the variety of vitamins and minerals that mixed veggies provide.

Soup with Lentils and Veggies

Preparation Time: 15 minutes .

Cooking Time: 30 minutes

Servings: 6

Ingredients:

- one cup of washed dry lentils
- Six cups of vegetable stock
- two chopped carrots
- two chopped celery stalks
- one sliced onion
- three minced garlic cloves
- One can of chopped tomatoes (14 ounces)
- A single tsp of dried thyme
- One tsp of dehydrated oregano
- One bay leaf
- Two tsp olive oil
- As a garnish, use fresh parsley.
- To taste, add salt and pepper.

Instructions:

- Warm up the olive oil in a big saucepan over medium heat. Add the diced carrots, celery, minced garlic, and onion. Cook the veggies until they start to become tender.
- To the saucepan, add the rinsed lentils, chopped tomatoes, vegetable broth, dried oregano, dry thyme, and bay leaf. Heat till boiling.

- Once the lentils are soft, reduce the heat to low, cover, and simmer for 25 to 30 minutes.
- Remove the bay leaf and add salt and pepper to taste.
- Before serving, garnish with fresh parsley.

Nutritional Value (Per Serving):

Approximately 160 calories, 9g of protein, 24g of carbohydrates, 4g of fat, 8g of fiber

Health Benefits:

1. Rich in Fiber and Protein: Rich in fiber and protein, lentils promote satiety and easy digestion.
2. Vitamin-Packed: The abundance of veggies in this soup provides a range of vitamins and minerals.

<u>Black bean and Quinoa Salad</u>

Preparation Time: 20 minutes

Servings: 4.

Ingredients:

- One cup of washed quinoa
- One can (15 ounces) of black beans, washed and drained
- One sliced red bell pepper
- Half a cup fresh, canned, or defrosted frozen corn kernels
- 1/4 cup of coarsely chopped red onion
- 1/4 cup finely chopped fresh cilantro
- two limes' worth of juice
- Two tsp olive oil
- One teaspoon of cumin powder
- To taste, add salt and pepper.
- Cuts of avocado to garnish (optional)

Instructions:

- To cook the quinoa, according to the package's instructions. After cooking, use a fork to fluff and let to cool.
- Cooked quinoa, black beans, sliced red onion, diced bell pepper, corn kernels, and fresh cilantro should all be combined in a big mixing dish.
- Mix the lime juice, olive oil, ground cumin, salt, and pepper in a separate small bowl.
- After adding the dressing to the quinoa mixture, toss to fully incorporate.
- If necessary, taste and adjust the seasoning.
- If preferred, garnish with avocado slices before to serving.

Nutritional Value (Per Serving):

Approximately 220 calories, 9g of protein, 33g of carbohydrates, 7g of fat, 8g of fiber

Health Benefits:

1. Rich in Protein and Fiber: Quinoa and black beans are also excellent sources of these nutrients.
2. Vitamin-Rich: There are so many different vitamins and minerals in this salad since it is so full of veggies.

Avocado and Chickpea Salad

Preparation Time: 15 minutes .

Servings: 4.

Ingredients:

- Two cans of washed and drained chickpeas, 15 ounces each
- two chopped avocados
- one chopped cucumber
- 1/4 cup of coarsely chopped red onion
- 1/4 cup finely chopped fresh parsley
- One lemon's juice
- Two tsp olive oil
- One teaspoon of cumin
- To taste, add salt and pepper.

Instructions:

- Chickpeas, diced avocados, diced cucumbers, sliced red onion, and fresh parsley should all be combined in a big mixing dish.
- Mix the lemon juice, olive oil, cumin, salt, and pepper in a separate small bowl.
- After adding the dressing to the salad, toss everything together well.
- If necessary, taste and adjust the seasoning.

Nutritional Value (Per Serving):

Approximately 280 calories, 9g of protein, 28g of carbohydrates, 15g of fat, 10g of fiber

Health Benefits:

1. Protein and excellent Fats: Chickpeas and avocado come together in this salad, which offers an excellent amount of both.
2. Rich in Nutrients: The components used in its preparation provide a wealth of fiber and other nutrients.

Quinoa Salad with Mediterranean Flavors

Preparation Time: 20 minutes

Servings: 4.

Ingredients:

- One cup of washed quinoa
- Half a cup of cherry tomatoes
- one chopped cucumber
- Sliced and pitted half a cup of Kalamata olives
- 1/4 cup of coarsely chopped red onion
- 1/4 cup finely chopped fresh parsley
- 1/4 cup finely chopped fresh mint leaves
- One lemon's juice
- Three tablespoons pure olive oil
- One tsp of dehydrated oregano
- To taste, add salt and pepper.
- Feta cheese crumbles (optional)

Instructions:

- To cook the quinoa, according to the package's instructions. After cooking, use a fork to fluff and let to cool.
- Cooked quinoa, diced cucumber, split cherry tomatoes, sliced Kalamata olives, chopped red onion, fresh parsley, and fresh mint leaves should all be combined in a big mixing basin.
- Mix the dried oregano, extra virgin olive oil, lemon juice, salt, and pepper in a separate small bowl.
- After adding the dressing to the salad, toss everything together well.
- If preferred, sprinkle some crumbled feta cheese on top before serving.

Nutritional Value (Per Serving):

Approximately 240 calories, 6g of protein, 28g of carbohydrates, 12g of fat, 5g of fiber

Health Benefits:

1. High in protein and nutrition: Quinoa provides a variety of nutrients, while the vegetables provide vitamins and minerals.
2. Mediterranean Flavors: Adding olives and olive oil to food gives it a distinctive Mediterranean taste and healthy fats.

Curry made with vegan chickpeas

Preparation Time: 15 minutes.

Cooking Time: 25 minutes

Servings: 4.

Ingredients:

- Two cans of washed and drained chickpeas, 15 ounces each
- One onion, chopped finely
- three minced garlic cloves
- One tablespoon of freshly grated ginger
- One can of chopped tomatoes (14 ounces)
- One 14-ounce can of coconut milk
- two cups of spinach leaves
- Curry powder, two teaspoons
- one tsp finely ground turmeric
- One teaspoon of cumin powder
- One tablespoon of coconut oil
- To taste, add salt and pepper.
- To garnish, use fresh cilantro.

Instructions:

- In a large pan set over medium heat, warm the coconut oil. Sauté the chopped onion until it becomes transparent.
- Add the grated ginger and minced garlic, and simmer for an additional minute, or until fragrant.
- Add the ground cumin, turmeric, and curry powder and stir. Cook for one to two minutes.
- Add the coconut milk, chickpeas, and chopped tomatoes. Simmer for ten minutes.
- After adding the fresh spinach, simmer it for a further five minutes, or until it wilts.
- Season with salt and pepper, to taste.
- Before serving, garnish with fresh cilantro.

Nutritional Value (Per Serving):

Approximately 260 calories, 10g of protein, 30g of carbohydrates, 12g of fat, Fiber: nine grams

Health Benefits:

1. Plant-Based Protein: Packed with protein from chickpeas, this curry is both filling and healthy.
2. Rich in Vitamins: By adding vitamins and minerals, spinach improves the nutritional profile of the food.

Lentil Shepherd's Pie for Vegans

Preparation Time: 15 minutes

Cooking Time: 40 minutes

Servings: 6

Ingredients:

Regarding the Filling:

- One cup of washed and dried brown or green lentils
- three cups of broth made from vegetables
- One chopped onion
- two chopped carrots
- two minced garlic cloves
- One cup of frozen peas
- One spoonful of pasted tomatoes
- A single tsp of dried thyme
- One tsp of dehydrated rosemary
- To taste, add salt and pepper.
- Two tsp olive oil

Regarding the Mashed Potato Garnish:

- Peel and dice four big potatoes.
- 1/4 cup plant-based milk, such as unsweetened almond milk
- Two tsp vegan butter
- To taste, add salt and pepper.

Instructions:

Regarding the Filling:

- Lentils and vegetable broth should be combined in a pot. Once the lentils are soft and the liquid has been absorbed, bring to a boil, lower the heat, and simmer for 20 to 25 minutes.
- The olive oil should be warmed over medium heat in a separate pan. Add the chopped garlic, carrots, and onion. Sauté the food until it becomes tender.
- To the onion and carrot combination, add cooked lentils, frozen peas, tomato paste, dried thyme, dried rosemary, salt, and pepper. Simmer for five more minutes. Put aside.

Regarding the Mashed Potato Garnish:

- In a saucepan of salted water, boil the diced potatoes until they become soft. Make sure to drain properly.
- While the potatoes are still warm, mash them. Stir in vegan butter, almond milk, salt, and pepper. Blend until a creamy, smooth consistency is achieved.
- Putting the Shepherd's Pie Together:
- Turn the oven on to 375°F, or 190°C.
- Spoon the lentil mixture over the vegetables in a baking dish.
- Evenly distribute the mashed potatoes on top of the lentil mixture.
- Bake for twenty to twenty-five minutes, or until golden brown on top.
- Warm up the food.

Nutritional Value (Per Serving):

Approximately 320 calories, 13g of protein, 52g of carbohydrates, 7g of fat, 11g of fiber

Health Benefits:

1. High in Protein and Fiber: Lentils provide protein and fiber to a diet, making it more balanced.
2. Minerals and Vitamins: The veggies and lentils in this recipe are a great source of vitamins.

Sandwich Filling: Chickpea Salad

Preparation Time: 15 minutes.

4-6 servings in total

Ingredients:

- Two cans of washed and drained chickpeas, 15 ounces each
- Half a cup of finely chopped celery
- 1/4 cup of coarsely chopped red onion
- 1/4 cup finely chopped fresh parsley
- 1/4 cup vegan mayonnaise
- One spoonful of mustard dijon
- One tablespoon of lemon juice
- half a teaspoon of powdered garlic
- To taste, add salt and pepper.
- Lettuce stems
- sandwich buns or sliced bread

Instructions:

- Using a fork or potato masher, mash the chickpeas in a mixing dish until they become chunky.
- To the mashed chickpeas, add finely chopped celery, red onion, and fresh parsley.
- Combine the vegan mayonnaise, Dijon mustard, lemon juice, garlic powder, salt, and pepper in a separate small bowl.
- After adding the dressing to the chickpea mixture, thoroughly mix it in.
- If necessary, taste and adjust the seasoning.
- Present the chickpea salad with lettuce leaves on sandwich rolls or slices of bread.

Nutritional Value (Per Serving):

Approximately 230 calories, 9g of protein, 28g of carbohydrates, 8g of fat, 8g of fiber

Health Benefits:

1. Rich in Protein: Chickpeas are a fantastic plant-based source of protein.
2. Fiber and Flavor: The herbs and veggies improve the flavor and provide fiber to the dish.

Black bean burger for vegans

Preparation Time: 20 minutes

Cooking Time: 10 minutes

Servings: 4.

Ingredients:

- Two cans (15 ounces each) of rinsed and drained black beans
- Half a cup of whole wheat or gluten-free bread crumbs
- 1/4 cup of coarsely chopped red onion
- 1/4 cup finely sliced bell peppers, any color
- two minced garlic cloves
- Two teaspoons of freshly cut cilantro
- One tablespoon of cumin powder
- One tsp of paprika
- To taste, add salt and pepper.
- Use olive oil for cooking.
- buns for burgers
- your preferred toppings (tomato, avocado, lettuce, etc.)

Instructions:

- Mash half of the black beans into a paste in a mixing basin. Leaving some whole beans for texture, add the remaining beans and gently mash.
- To the mashed beans, add bread crumbs, diced red onion, chopped bell peppers, minced

garlic, fresh cilantro, paprika, ground cumin, and salt and pepper. Blend until well blended.

- Separate the ingredients into four equal parts and form each into a burger pattin.
- In a pan over medium heat, warm the olive oil. Cook the patties until a golden crust forms, about 4–5 minutes each side.
- Top the black bean burgers with your preferred toppings and serve them on burger buns.

Value for Nutrition (per serving, excluding bread and toppings):

Approximately 230 calories, 13g of protein, 38g of carbohydrates, Fat (2 grams), 13g of fiber

Health Benefits:

1. Rich in Protein and Fiber: Black beans are a strong source of both.
2. Minimal Fat: When compared to conventional meat-based burgers, this vegan burger has less fat.

Wraps with Vegan Chickpea Salad

Preparation Time: 15 minutes.

Servings: 4 (each wraps).

Ingredients:

- One can (15 ounces) of rinsed and drained chickpeas
- 1/4 cup vegan mayonnaise
- two tsp lemon juice
- 1/4 cup of coarsely chopped red onion

- 1/4 cup finely chopped celery
- Two teaspoons of freshly chopped parsley
- To taste, add salt and pepper.
- Four substantial whole-grain wraps
- Spinach or lettuce leaves for assembling
- Avocado and tomato slices for the stuffing

Instructions:

- To partly mash the chickpeas, use a fork or potato masher in a mixing basin.
- To the mashed chickpeas, add vegan mayonnaise, lemon juice, red onion, celery, and fresh parsley. Toss to blend thoroughly.
- To taste, add more salt and pepper to the mixture.
- Arrange the whole grain wrappers in a tidy manner. Put some spinach or lettuce leaves in the middle of each wrapper.
- Spoon the chickpea salad evenly over the spinach or lettuce leaves in each wrapper.
- Place avocado and tomato slices over the chickpea salad.
- The wraps should be securely rolled once the sides are folded toward the center.
- Once each wrap is diagonally cut in half, scrve.

Nutritional Value (per wrap, per serving):

Approximately 280 calories, 10g of protein, 40g of carbohydrates, 9g of fat, 8g of fiber

Health Benefits:

1. Protein and Fiber: Chickpeas are a fantastic source of both protein and fiber, which help with digestion and satiety.
2. Minerals and vitamins: Various vitamins and minerals may be found in foods including parsley, celery, and red onions.

Vegan Curry with Chickpeas and Eggplant

Preparation Time: 20 minutes

Cooking Time: 25 minutes

Servings: 4.

Ingredients:

- One big sliced eggplant
- One can (15 ounces) of rinsed and drained chickpeas
- One onion, chopped finely
- three minced garlic cloves
- one-inch-long, grated ginger slice
- One can of chopped tomatoes (14 ounces)
- One 14-ounce can of coconut milk
- Curry powder, two teaspoons
- One teaspoon of cumin powder
- One tsp finely ground coriander
- One tsp of turmeric
- One tablespoon of olive oil
- To taste, add salt and pepper.
- To garnish, use fresh cilantro.

Instructions:

- In a big skillet or pan, warm up the olive oil over medium heat. Sauté the chopped onion until it becomes transparent.
- Add the grated ginger and minced garlic, and simmer for

an additional minute, or until fragrant.

- Cook for one to two minutes after adding the curry powder, powdered cumin, ground coriander, and turmeric.
- Stir to coat the chickpeas and chopped eggplant with the spices in the pan.
- Add the coconut milk and chopped tomatoes. Simmer until the eggplant is soft and the curry has thickened, about 15 to 20 minutes.
- Season with salt and pepper, to taste.
- Before serving, garnish with fresh cilantro.

Nutritional Value (Per Serving):

Approximately 260 calories, 9g of protein, 28g of carbohydrates, 13g of fat, 11g of fiber

Health Benefits:

1. High in Fiber and Flavor: The combination of eggplant and chickpeas in this curry gives it a flavorful kick from the spices as well as fiber.
2. Plant-based protein can be found in chickpeas, which makes them a fantastic vegan option.

Pasta with Cherry Tomato and Asparagus

Preparation Time: 20 minutes

Cooking Time: 15 minutes

Servings: 4.

Ingredients:

- Eight ounces of your favorite pasta, or whole wheat spaghetti

- One bunch of asparagus, thinly sliced into 1-inch segments
- One pint of halved cherry tomatoes
- three minced garlic cloves
- 1/4 cup finely chopped fresh basil leaves
- Two tsp olive oil
- One lemon's juice
- one lemon's zest
- To taste, add salt and pepper.
- For serving, grated Parmesan cheese or nutritional yeast (optional)

Instructions:

- Boil the pasta in salted water until al dente, following the directions on the box. With the exception of roughly 1/2 cup of pasta water, drain and put aside.
- Heat the olive oil in a big pan over medium heat while the pasta cooks. Cook the minced garlic for one minute, or until it becomes aromatic.
- When the asparagus pieces begin to soften, add them to the pan and sauté them for three to four minutes.
- When the cherry tomatoes begin to soften, add them to the skillet and simmer for a further two to three minutes.
- Add the chopped basil, lemon zest, cooked pasta, and lemon juice. Mix everything until well incorporated. To loosen the pasta, add a little amount of the leftover pasta water if necessary.
- Season with salt and pepper, to taste.
- Serve the pasta with asparagus and cherry tomatoes with nutritional yeast or optionally, grated Parmesan cheese.

Value of Nutrition (Approximately for Each Serving):

Approximately 300 calories, 9g of protein, 50g of carbohydrates, 8g of fat, 8g of fiber

Health Benefits:

1. Nutrition of Asparagus: Asparagus has a significant quantity of fiber and is high in folate, vitamins A, C, and K.
2. Cherry Tomatoes: Rich in nutrients but low in calories, cherry tomatoes include antioxidants like lycopene.

Brussels sprouts roasted in a balsamic glaze

Preparation Time: 10 minutes

Cooking Time: 25 minutes

Servings: 4.

Ingredients:

- One pound of halved and trimmed Brussels sprouts
- Two tsp olive oil
- To taste, add salt and pepper.
- Two teaspoons of homemade or store-bought balsamic glaze
- Optional garnishes include nutritional yeast or grated Parmesan cheese.

Instructions:

- Adjust the oven temperature to 400°F (200°C) and place parchment paper on a baking pan.
- Toss the halved Brussels sprouts with olive oil, salt, and pepper in a mixing dish until well coated.

- Arrange the Brussels sprouts on the baking sheet that has been preheated in a single layer.
- Once the oven is warmed, roast the Brussels sprouts for 20 to 25 minutes, tossing them halfway through, or until they become soft when probed with a fork and become golden brown.
- After taking the roasted Brussels sprouts out of the oven, place them on a platter for serving.
- After lightly tossing to ensure uniform coating, drizzle the roasted Brussels sprouts with the balsamic glaze.
- If preferred, top the roasted Brussels sprouts with a little nutritional yeast or grated Parmesan cheese.

Value of Nutrition (Approximately for Each Serving):

Approximately 100 calories, 3g of protein, 10g of carbohydrates, 6g of fat, 4g of fiber

Health Benefits:

1. Nutritional Value of Brussels Sprouts: High in fiber, antioxidants, and vitamins K and C.
2. Balsamic Glaze: A lower-calorie substitute for heavier sauces, the balsamic glaze offers a tangy sweetness.

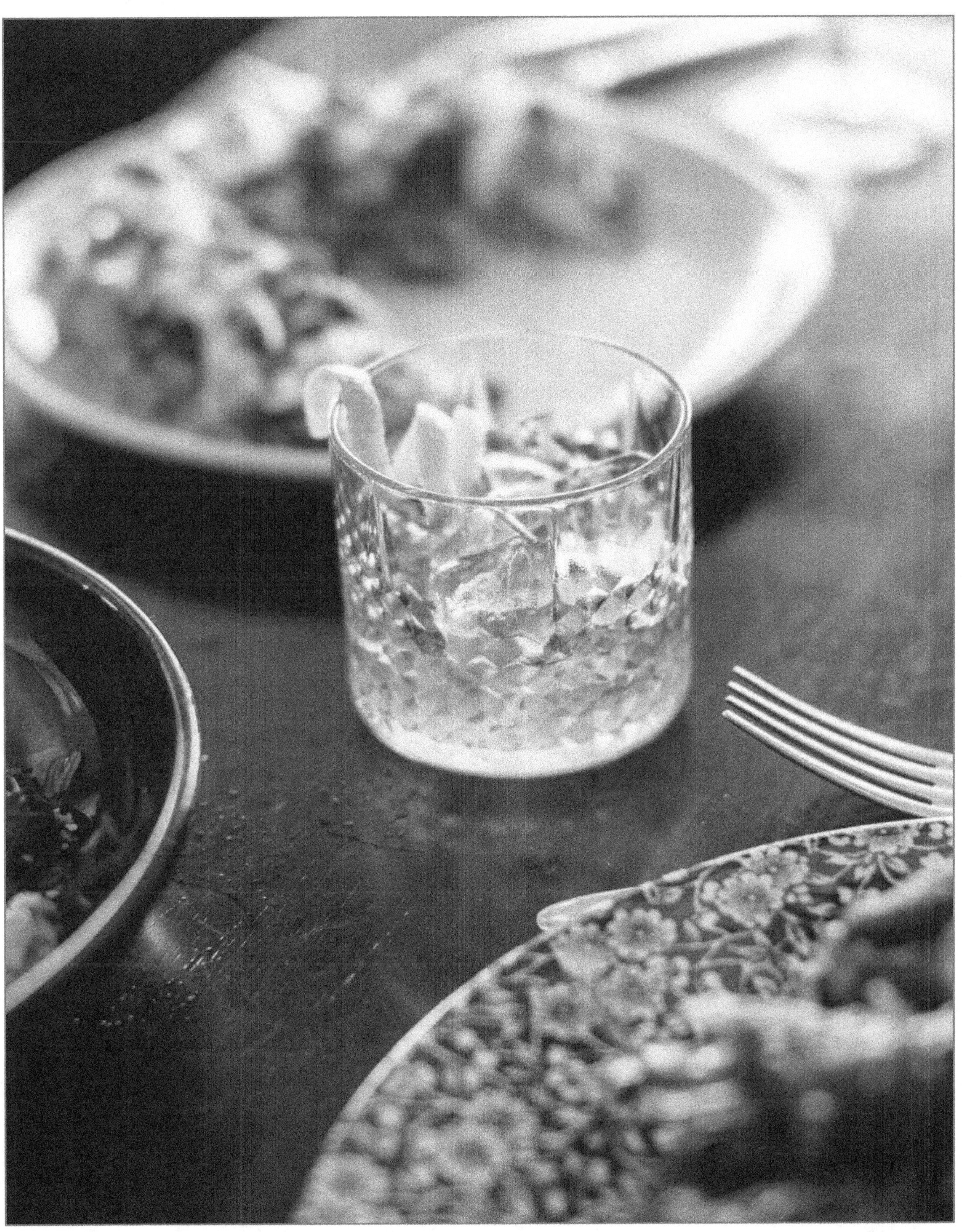

05

Black Bean Soup

Preparation Time: 15 minutes

Cooking Time: 30 minutes

Servings: 6

Ingredients:

- 2 cups dried black beans, soaked overnight
- 1 onion, finely chopped
- 2 cloves garlic, minced
- 2 carrots, diced
- 2 celery stalks, diced
- 1 red bell pepper, diced
- 4 cups low-sodium vegetable broth
- 1 can (14 oz) diced tomatoes
- 1 teaspoon cumin
- 1 teaspoon smoked paprika
- Salt and pepper to taste
- Chopped fresh cilantro for garnish

Instructions:

- Soak Beans: Rinse and soak black beans overnight. Drain and rinse before use.
- Sauté Aromatics: In a pot, sauté onion and garlic until fragrant. Add carrots, celery, and bell

pepper. Cook until slightly softened.

- Simmer Soup: Add soaked black beans, vegetable broth, diced tomatoes, cumin, and smoked paprika. Bring to a boil, then reduce heat and simmer for 30 minutes or until beans are tender.

- Season and Serve: Season with salt and pepper. Garnish with chopped cilantro before serving.

Nutritional Value (Per Serving - 1 cup):

Calories: 220, Protein: 12g, Carbohydrates: 40g, Fat: 1g, Fiber: 10g

Health Benefits and Nutritional Insights:

1. High in Fiber: Black beans are rich in fiber, aiding in digestion and promoting fullness.
2. Plant-Based Protein: Provides a good source of plant-based protein.
3. Low in Fat: A low-fat option packed with nutrients.

Tomato Basil Soup

Preparation Time: 10 minutes

Cooking Time: 25 minutes

Servings: 4

Ingredients:

- 6 large tomatoes, diced
- 1 onion, chopped
- 3 cloves garlic, minced
- 4 cups low-sodium vegetable broth

- ½ cup chopped fresh basil leaves

- Salt and pepper to taste

Instructions:

- In a pot, sauté onions and garlic until translucent.

- Add diced tomatoes and vegetable broth. After bringing to a boil, simmer for twenty minutes.

- Stir in fresh basil leaves and let it simmer for an additional 5 minutes.

- Blend the soup until smooth using an immersion blender or by transferring it to a regular blender.

- To taste, adjust the salt and pepper.

Nutritional Value (Per Serving - approximately 1.5 cups):

Calories: 60, Protein: 2g, Carbohydrates: 14g, Fat: 1g, Fiber: 4g

Health Benefits and Nutritional Insights:

1. Low-Calorie, High Fiber: Tomato and basil soup is low in calories and high in fiber, aiding in digestion.

2. Vitamins and Antioxidants: Tomatoes and basil provide essential vitamins and antioxidants.

Chicken Vegetable Soup

Preparation Time: 15 minutes

Cooking Time: 30 minutes

Servings: 6

Ingredients:

- 1 lb chicken breast, diced

- 1 cup diced carrots

- 1 cup diced celery

- 1 cup diced onions
- 1 cup chopped tomatoes
- 1 cup corn kernels
- 8 cups low-sodium chicken broth
- 2 cloves garlic, minced
- 1 tablespoon olive oil
- Salt and pepper to taste
- Fresh parsley for garnish

Instructions:

- Warm up the olive oil in a saucepan over medium heat. Sauté diced chicken until lightly browned. Remove chicken and set aside.
- Add the celery, carrots, and onions to the same saucepan.. Sauté until they begin to soften, then add minced garlic. Cook for another minute.
- Add diced tomatoes, corn kernels, sautéed chicken, and chicken broth. Heat to a boil, then simmer for 20 to 25 minutes on low heat..
- Season with salt and pepper to taste. Garnish with fresh parsley before serving.

Nutritional Value (Per Serving)::

Calories: 180, Protein: 20g, Carbohydrates: 15g, Fat: 4g, Fiber: 3g

Health Benefits and Nutritional Insights:

1. Lean Protein: Chicken offers lean protein, aiding in muscle maintenance.
2. Vegetable Nutrients: Carrots, celery, and tomatoes provide vitamins and antioxidants.

<u>**Butternut Squash Soup**</u>

Preparation Time: 15 minutes

Cooking Time: 30 minutes

Servings: 4

Ingredients:

- 1 medium butternut squash, peeled and diced (about 4 cups)
- Chopped onions, carrots, celery (1 cup each)
- Low-sodium vegetable broth (4 cups)
- Minced garlic (2 cloves)
- Fresh thyme or dried thyme (1 teaspoon)
- Salt and pepper to taste

Instructions:

- Saute the celery, carrots, and onions in a saucepan until they are tender. Grated garlic is added and cooked for one minute.
- Add diced butternut squash, vegetable broth, thyme, salt, and pepper. Once the squash is soft, lower heat and simmer for 20 to 25 minutes after bringing to a boil.
- Using an immersion blender, grind the soup until they're smooth.

Nutritional Value (Per Serving - 1.5 cups):

Calories: 80, Protein: 2g, Carbohydrates: 20g, Fat: 0.5g, Fiber: 5g

Health Benefits and Nutritional Insights:

1. High in Vitamins: Butternut squash is rich in vitamin A, C, and other nutrients.

2. Low-Calorie: This soup is low in calories and high in fiber, making it a healthy and filling option.

Minestrone Soup

Preparation Time: 15 minutes

Cooking Time: 30 minutes

Servings: 6

Ingredients:

- 1 tablespoon olive oil
- 1 onion, diced (1 cup)
- 2 carrots, diced (1 cup)
- 2 celery stalks, diced (1 cup)
- 3 cloves garlic, minced
- 1 can (14 oz) diced tomatoes
- 6 cups low-sodium vegetable broth
- One can (15 oz) of washed and drained kidney beans
- 1 cup chopped green beans
- One cup of little pasta, such shells or ditalini
- 2 cups chopped spinach or kale
- 1 teaspoon dried oregano
- 1 teaspoon dried basil
- Salt and pepper to taste
- Grated Parmesan cheese for garnish (optional)

Instructions:

- Heat olive oil in a large pot over medium heat. Add diced onions, carrots, and celery. Let the veggies soften by sautéing them for 5 to 7 minutes.
- Once again, sauté for one minute after adding the minced garlic..
- Pour in diced tomatoes and vegetable broth. Bring to a boil.

- Stir in kidney beans, green beans, and pasta. When pasta is al dente, simmer for ten to twelve minutes.

- Add chopped spinach or kale, dried oregano, dried basil, salt, and pepper. Simmer for an additional 5 minutes.

- Serve hot, optionally garnishing with grated Parmesan cheese.

Nutritional Value (Per Serving)::

Calories: 200, Protein: 9g, Carbohydrates: 35g, Fat: 3g, Fiber: 8g

Health Benefits and Nutritional Insights:

1. High in Fiber: Loaded with vegetables and beans, providing a good amount of fiber.
2. Nutrient-Rich: Packed with vitamins and minerals from the variety of vegetables.

Vegetable Lentil Soup

Preparation Time: 15 minutes

Cooking Time: 30 minutes

Servings: 6

Ingredients:

- 1 cup dried lentils, rinsed
- 1 cup chopped onions
- 1 cup chopped carrots
- 1 cup chopped celery
- 4 cups low-sodium vegetable broth
- 2 cups diced tomatoes
- 2 cloves minced garlic
- 1 teaspoon dried thyme
- 1 teaspoon dried oregano
- Salt and pepper to taste

Instructions:

- Saute the celery, carrots, and onions in a saucepan until they are tender.
- Add the chopped garlic and cook it for one minute.
- Add lentils, vegetable broth, diced tomatoes, dried thyme, dried oregano, salt, and pepper. Bring to a boil, then simmer for 25-30 minutes or until lentils are tender.

Nutritional Value (Per Serving)::

Calories: 180, Protein: 12g, Carbohydrates: 32g, Fat: 1g, Fiber: 10g

Health Benefits and Nutritional Insights:

1. High in Protein and Fiber: Lentils are rich in both protein and fiber, aiding in satiety and digestion.

2. Low in Fat: This soup is low in fat and provides essential nutrients from vegetables and lentils.

Turkey and Vegetable Stew

Preparation Time: 15 minutes

Cooking Time: 35 minutes

Servings: 6

Ingredients:

- 1 lb lean ground turkey
- 1 cup chopped onions
- 1 cup chopped carrots
- 1 cup chopped celery
- 2 cloves garlic, minced
- 4 cups low-sodium chicken broth
- 1 can (14 oz) diced tomatoes
- 2 cups chopped zucchini

- 2 cups frozen green beans
- 2 bay leaves
- 1 teaspoon dried thyme
- Salt and pepper to taste

Instructions:

- In a pot, brown the lean ground turkey over medium heat until no longer pink. Add onions, carrots, celery, and garlic. Sauté until vegetables soften.
- Add chicken broth, diced tomatoes, zucchini, frozen green beans, bay leaves, dried thyme, salt, and pepper. After reaching a boil, lower the heat, and simmer for 25 to 30 minutes.
- Remove bay leaves before serving.

Nutritional Value (Per Serving)::

Calories: 180, Protein: 20g, Carbohydrates: 12g, Fat: 5g, Fiber: 4g

Health Benefits and Nutritional Insights:

1. Lean Protein Source: Turkey provides lean protein, supporting muscle health.
2. Vegetable-Rich: Packed with vegetables, offering essential vitamins and minerals.

Quinoa Vegetable Soup

Preparation Time: 15 minutes

Cooking Time: 30 minutes

Servings: 6

Ingredients:

- 1 cup quinoa, rinsed
- Chopped onions, carrots, celery
- Low-sodium vegetable broth
- Diced tomatoes
- Chopped zucchini

- Minced garlic

- Fresh thyme

- Salt and pepper to taste

- Chopped fresh parsley for garnish

Instructions:

- In a pot, sauté onions, carrots, celery, and minced garlic until softened.

- Add diced tomatoes, chopped zucchini, vegetable broth, fresh thyme, salt, and pepper. Bring to a boil.

- Add rinsed quinoa to the boiling mixture. Reduce heat, cover, and simmer for 15-20 minutes or until quinoa is cooked and vegetables are tender.

- Serve hot, garnished with chopped fresh parsley.

Nutritional Value (Per Serving - one & half cups):

Calories: 150, Protein: 6g, Carbohydrates: 28g, Fat: 2g, Fiber: 5g

Health Benefits and Nutritional Insights:

1. High in Protein and Fiber: Quinoa provides complete protein while vegetables offer fiber and essential nutrients.

2. Balanced Nutrition: This soup is well-balanced, providing a variety of vitamins and minerals.

Spicy Chickpea Stew

Preparation Time: 15 minutes

Cooking Time: 30 minutes

Servings: 4

Ingredients:

- 2 cans (15 oz each) chickpeas, drained and rinsed
- Chopped onions, bell peppers, tomatoes
- Minced garlic
- Low-sodium vegetable broth
- Tomato paste (2 tablespoons)
- Smoked paprika (1 teaspoon)
- Cumin (1 teaspoon)
- Chili powder (1/2 teaspoon)
- Red pepper flakes (1/4 teaspoon, optional)
- Salt and pepper to taste
- Fresh cilantro for garnish

Instructions:

- In a pot, sauté onions, bell peppers, and garlic until softened.
- Add chickpeas, chopped tomatoes, tomato paste, vegetable broth, smoked paprika, cumin, chili powder, red pepper flakes (if using), salt, and pepper. Cook for 20 to 25 minutes after bringing to a simmer.
- Adjust seasoning to taste and simmer for another 5 minutes.
- Serve hot, garnished with fresh cilantro.

Nutritional Value (Per Serving)::

Calories: 180, Protein: 8g, Carbohydrates: 30g, Fat: 2g, Fiber: 8g

Health Benefits and Nutritional Insights:

1. Rich in Protein and Fiber: Chickpeas are high in both protein and fiber, aiding in satiety and digestive health.
2. Low in Fat: This stew is low in fat and offers essential nutrients from vegetables and legumes.

Broccoli and Cheese Soup

Preparation Time: 10 minutes

Cooking Time: 25 minutes

Servings: 4

Ingredients:

- 4 cups chopped broccoli florets
- 1 small onion, finely chopped
- 2 cloves garlic, minced
- 4 cups low-sodium vegetable broth
- 1 cup low-fat milk
- 1 cup low-fat shredded cheddar cheese
- 2 tablespoons cornstarch
- Salt and pepper to taste

Instructions:

- In a pot, sauté onions and garlic until translucent. Add chopped broccoli and sauté for a few minutes.
- Add the veggie broth and heat until it boils. Reduce heat and simmer for 15-20 minutes until broccoli is tender.
- In a small bowl, mix cornstarch with a bit of water to create a slurry. Stir the slurry into the soup and simmer for a few minutes until slightly thickened.
- Reduce heat to low. Stir in low-fat milk and shredded cheddar cheese until the cheese is melted and the soup is heated through. Be careful not to boil.
- Season with salt and pepper to taste.

Nutritional Value (Per Serving)::

Calories: 150, Protein: 10g, Carbohydrates: 15g, Fat: 5g, Fiber: 4g

Health Benefits and Nutritional Insights:

1. Low-Fat Dairy: The use of low-fat cheese reduces fat content while providing calcium and protein.
2. High in Vitamins: Broccoli is rich in vitamins and antioxidants, promoting overall health.

Mushroom Barley Soup

Time: 15 minutes

Cooking Time: 45 minutes

Servings: 6

Ingredients:

- 1 cup pearl barley, rinsed
- Sliced mushrooms (8 oz)
- Chopped onions (1 cup)
- Minced garlic (2 cloves)
- Low-sodium vegetable broth (6 cups)
- Chopped carrots (1 cup)
- Chopped celery (1 cup)
- Bay leaves (2)
- Fresh thyme (1 tablespoon)
- Salt and pepper to taste
- Chopped parsley for garnish

Instructions:

- In a pot, sauté onions, garlic, mushrooms, carrots, and celery until softened.
- Add vegetable broth, pearl barley, bay leaves, fresh thyme, salt, and pepper. Bring to a boil, then reduce heat and simmer for 35-40 minutes or until barley is tender.
- Remove bay leaves before serving.

- Garnish with chopped parsley.

Nutritional Value (Per Serving)::

Calories: 180, Protein: 6g, Carbohydrates: 38g, Fat: 1g, Fiber: 8g

Health Benefits and Nutritional Insights:

1. Rich in Fiber: Barley and vegetables contribute to the soup's fiber content, aiding in digestion and promoting fullness.
2. Low in Fat: This soup is low in fat and offers a good balance of carbohydrates and protein.

Cabbage and White Bean Soup

Preparation Time: 15 minutes

Cooking Time: 30 minutes

Servings: 4

Ingredients:

- 1 small head of cabbage, shredded
- One fifteen-ounce bag of washed and drained white beans
- Chopped onions, carrots, celery
- Low-sodium vegetable broth
- Minced garlic
- Bay leaves
- Thyme (fresh or dried)
- Salt and pepper to taste
- Chopped parsley for garnish

Instructions:

- In a pot, sauté onions, carrots, celery, and garlic until softened. Add shredded cabbage and cook for a few minutes until slightly wilted.
- Stir in white beans, vegetable broth, bay leaves, thyme, salt, and pepper. After bringing to a

boil, simmer for 20 to 25 minutes.

- Remove bay leaves before serving. Garnish with chopped parsley.

Nutritional Value (Per Serving)::

Calories: 120, Protein: 6g, Carbohydrates: 22g, Fat: 1g, Fiber: 8g

Health Benefits and Nutritional Insights:

1. High Fiber Content: Cabbage and white beans contribute to the fiber content, aiding in digestion and promoting satiety.
2. Low in Fat: This soup is low in fat and offers essential nutrients from vegetables and beans.

Lentil and Spinach Soup

Preparation Time: 10 minutes

Cooking Time: 25 minutes

Servings: 4

Ingredients:

- 1 cup dried lentils, rinsed
- Chopped onions (1 medium)
- Minced garlic (2 cloves)
- Low-sodium vegetable broth (4 cups)
- Diced tomatoes (1 can, 14 oz)
- Chopped spinach (2 cups)
- Bay leaves (2)
- Cumin (1 teaspoon)
- Salt and pepper to taste

Instructions:

- Simmer onions and garlic in a saucepan until they become tender. Stir for a minute after adding the washed lentils.

- Pour in vegetable broth, add diced tomatoes, bay leaves, cumin, salt, and pepper. Bring to a boil.

- Reduce heat and simmer for 20-25 minutes or until lentils are tender.

- Stir in chopped spinach and cook for an additional 3-5 minutes until wilted.

- Remove bay leaves before serving.

Nutritional Value (Per Serving):

Calories: 220, Protein: 15g, Carbohydrates: 40g, Fat: 1g, Fiber: 15g

Health Benefits and Nutritional Insights:

1. High in Protein and Fiber: Lentils provide a rich source of both protein and fiber, aiding in satiety and digestive health.

2. Low in Fat: This soup is low in fat and offers essential nutrients from lentils and spinach.

Carrot Ginger Soup

Preparation Time: 10 minutes

Cooking Time: 25 minutes

Servings: 4

Ingredients:

- 1pound carrots, peeled and chopped

- 1 small onion, chopped

- 2 cloves garlic, minced

- 1 tablespoon fresh ginger, grated

- 4 cups low-sodium vegetable broth

- Salt and pepper to taste
- Fresh cilantro for garnish (optional)

Instructions:

- In a pot, sauté chopped onions and garlic until translucent. Cook for a minute after adding the grated ginger.
- Add chopped carrots and vegetable broth. Bring to a boil, then reduce heat and simmer for 20-25 minutes or until carrots are tender.
- Using an immersion blender, puree the soup until it's completely smooth Alternatively, transfer the mixture to a blender and puree in batches until smooth.
- Season with salt and pepper to taste.

- Serve hot, garnished with fresh cilantro if desired.

Nutritional Value (Per Serving):

Calories: 80, Protein: 2g, Carbohydrates: 18g, Fat: 0.5g, Fiber: 4g

Health Benefits and Nutritional Insights:

1. Rich in Vitamin A: Carrots are a great source of vitamin A, promoting eye health.
2. Ginger's Health Benefits: Ginger possesses anti-inflammatory and antioxidant properties, contributing to overall health.

Spinach and Tomato Soup

Preparation Time: 10 minutes

Cooking Time: 20 minutes

Servings: 4

Ingredients:

- 1 can (400g) diced tomatoes
- 4 cups fresh spinach leaves
- 1 onion, chopped
- 2 cloves garlic, minced
- 4 cups low-sodium vegetable broth
- 1 teaspoon olive oil
- Salt and pepper to taste
- Fresh basil for garnish

Instructions:

- Heat olive oil in a pot. Add chopped onion and minced garlic. Sauté until the onion turns translucent.
- Add the diced tomatoes (including the juice from the can) to the pot and cook for 5 minutes.
- Pour in the vegetable broth and bring the mixture to a gentle boil. Simmer for an additional 10 minutes.
- Stir in the fresh spinach leaves and cook until wilted.
- To taste, adjust the salt and pepper.
- Serve hot, garnished with fresh basil leaves.

Nutritional Value (Per Serving)::

Calories: 60, Protein: 3g, Carbohydrates: 10g, Fat: 1g, Fiber: 3g

Health Benefits and Nutritional Insights:

1. Rich in Antioxidants: Spinach and tomatoes are packed with antioxidants and vitamins, supporting overall health.

2. Low-Calorie and Nutrient-Dense: This soup is low in calories but high in essential nutrients.

Curried Cauliflower Soup

Preparation Time: 10 minutes

Cooking Time: 25 minutes

Servings: 4

Ingredients:

- 1 medium head cauliflower, chopped
- 1 onion, chopped
- 2 cloves garlic, minced
- 4 cups low-sodium vegetable broth
- 1 teaspoon curry powder
- 1 teaspoon ground turmeric
- 1 teaspoon ground cumin
- Salt and pepper to taste
- Fresh cilantro for garnish

Instructions:

- Sauté garlic and onions in a saucepan until they become tender.
- Add chopped cauliflower, vegetable broth, curry powder, turmeric, and cumin. Bring to a boil, then reduce heat and simmer for 20 minutes or until cauliflower is tender.
- Puree the soup until it's smooth using an immersion blender or a blender.
- Season with salt and pepper to taste.
- Serve hot, garnished with fresh cilantro.

Nutritional Value (Per Serving)::

Calories: 70, Protein: 3g

Carbohydrates: 14g, Fat: 0.5g, Fiber: 5g

Health Benefits and Nutritional Insights:

1. Nutrient-Rich: Cauliflower is rich in vitamins C and K and provides fiber.
2. Low-Calorie and Low-Fat: This soup is low in calories and fat, making it a healthy choice.

Pea and Mint Soup

Preparation Time: 10 minutes

Cooking Time: 15 minutes

Servings: 4

Ingredients:

- 4 cups frozen peas
- 1 onion, chopped
- 4 cups low-sodium vegetable broth
- 2 tablespoons fresh mint leaves, chopped
- 2 cloves garlic, minced
- Salt and pepper to taste

Instructions:

- In a pot, sauté the chopped onion and garlic until the onion turns translucent.
- Add the frozen peas and vegetable broth. After bringing to a boil, lower the heat, and simmer for ten minutes or so.
- Stir in the fresh mint leaves and cook for an additional 2-3 minutes.
- Blend the soup until smooth, either with an immersion blender or by transferring it to a blender.

- To taste, adjust the salt and pepper.

Nutritional Value (Per Serving)::

Calories: 90, Protein: 5g, Carbohydrates: 15g, Fat: 1g, Fiber: 5g

Health Benefits and Nutritional Insights:

1. High in Fiber: Peas are rich in fiber, aiding in digestion and promoting a feeling of fullness.
2. Low-Calorie, High Nutrient Density: This soup is low in calories but packed with nutrients from peas and fresh mint.

Sweet Potato and Kale Stew

Preparation Time: 15 minutes

Cooking Time: 25 minutes

Servings: 6

Ingredients:

- 3 medium sweet potatoes, peeled and diced
- 1 bunch kale, stems removed and chopped
- 1 onion, finely chopped
- 4 cups low-sodium vegetable broth
- 3 cloves garlic, minced
- 1 teaspoon paprika
- 1 teaspoon cumin
- Salt and pepper to taste
- Chopped fresh parsley for garnish

Instructions:

- Add the garlic and onions to a large saucepan and sauté until softened.

- Add diced sweet potatoes, chopped kale, vegetable broth, paprika, and cumin to the pot. Bring to a boil.

- The sweet potatoes should be simmered for 20 to 25 minutes, or until they are soft.

- Season with salt and pepper to taste.

- Serve hot, garnished with chopped fresh parsley.

Nutritional Value (Per Serving):

Calories: 120, Protein: 3g, Carbohydrates: 28g, Fat: 0.5g, Fiber: 5g

Health Benefits and Nutritional Insights:

Nutrient-Dense: Sweet potatoes are rich in vitamins, while kale provides essential nutrients.

Low in Fat: This stew is low in fat and offers a blend of flavors and nutrients.

Red Lentil Curry Soup

Preparation Time: 10 minutes

Cooking Time: 25 minutes

Servings: 4

Ingredients:

- 1 cup red lentils, rinsed
- Chopped onions (1/2 cup)
- Minced garlic (2 cloves)
- Chopped tomatoes (1 cup)
- Low-sodium vegetable broth (4 cups)
- Curry powder (2 teaspoons)
- Ground turmeric (1 teaspoon)
- Ground cumin (1 teaspoon)
- Salt and pepper to taste
- Chopped cilantro for garnish

Instructions:

- In a pot, sauté onions and garlic until onions are translucent.
- Add chopped tomatoes and cook for 2-3 minutes.
- Stir in red lentils, vegetable broth, curry powder, turmeric, and cumin. After bringing to a boil, simmer the lentils for 20 minutes, or until they become soft.
- Season with salt and pepper.
- Serve hot, garnished with chopped cilantro.

Nutritional Value (Per Serving)::

Calories: 200, Protein: 15g, Carbohydrates: 35g, Fat: 1g, Fiber: 15g

Health Benefits and Nutritional Insights:

1. High in Protein and Fiber: Red lentils are rich in protein and fiber, aiding in satiety and digestive health.
2. Low in Fat: This soup is low in fat and provides essential nutrients from lentils and spices.

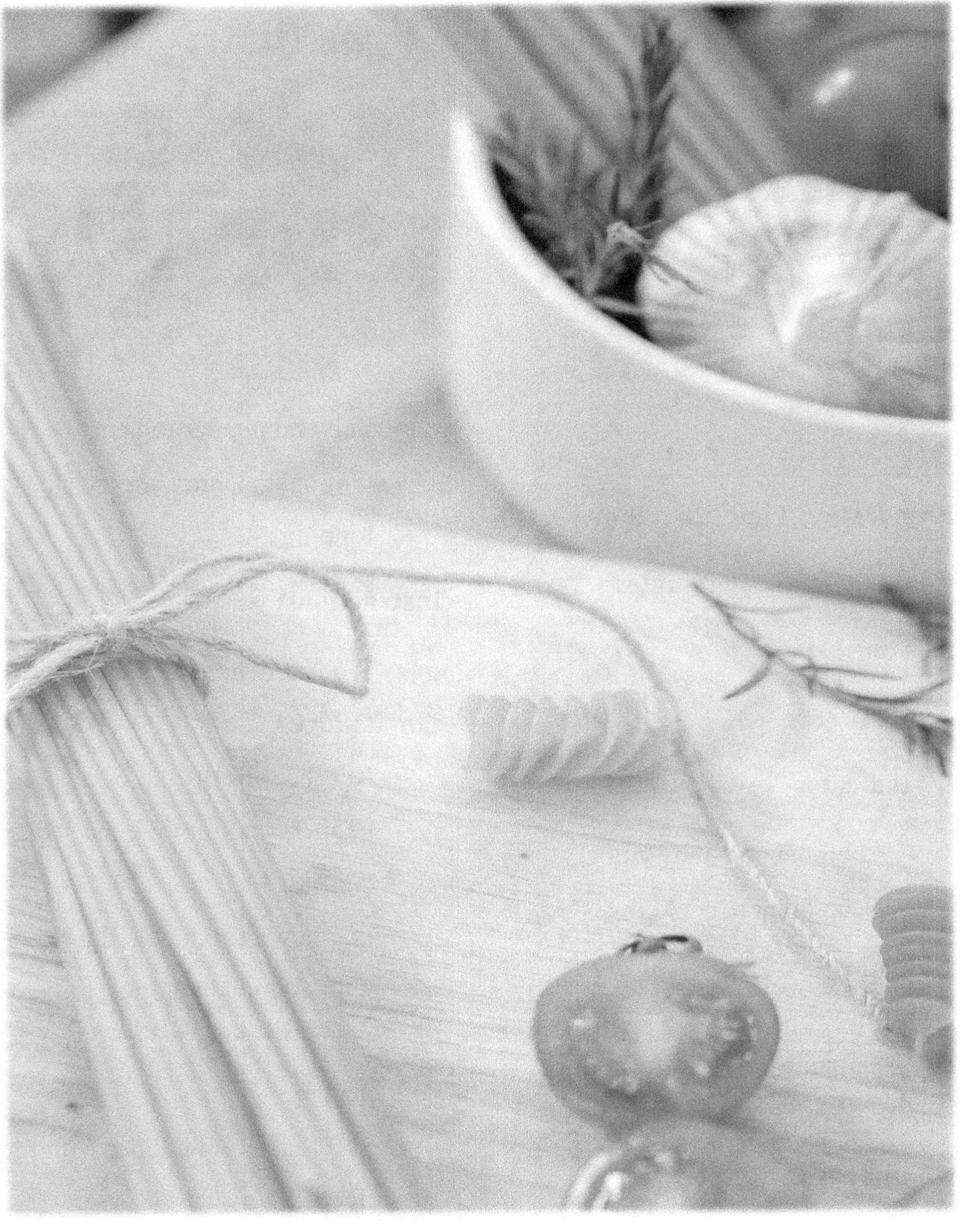

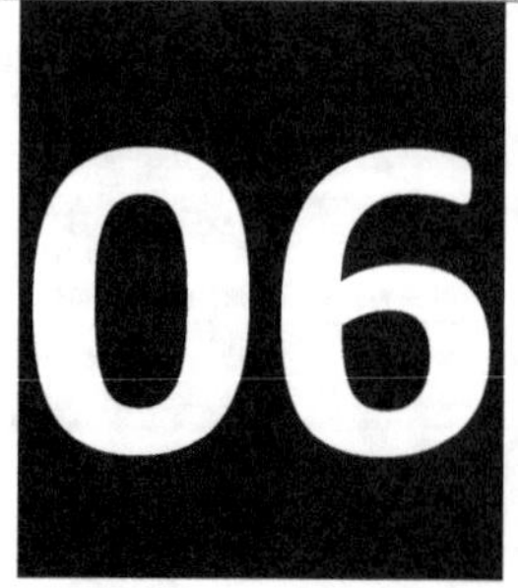

Quinoa-Stuffed Bell Peppers

Preparation Time: 20 minutes

Cooking Time: 40 minutes

Servings: 4

Ingredients:

- 4 bell peppers (any color)
- 1 cup quinoa, cooked
- Chopped veggies (such as onions, carrots, zucchini)
- Tomato sauce (low-sodium)
- Fresh greens (such as parsley or basil)
- Salt and pepper to taste
- Optional: Vegan cheese (for topping)

Instructions:

- Preheat oven to 375°F (190°C).
- Cut the tops off the bell peppers and remove the seeds and skins.
- In a bowl, mix cooked rice with chopped veggies, tomato sauce, fresh herbs, salt, and pepper.
- Stuff each bell pepper with the rice filling.

- Place the stuffed peppers in a baking dish. For 30 to 35 minutes, bake with a foil cover on.
- Remove the paper, add alternative vegan cheese on top, and bake for an additional 5 minutes until cheese melts.

Nutritional Value (Per Serving)::

Calories: Approximately 150, Protein: 5g, Carbohydrates: 30g, Fat: 1g, Fiber: 7g

Health Benefits and Nutritional Insights:

1. High in Fiber and Protein: Quinoa offers protein and fiber, helping in fullness and absorption.
2. Low-Calorie and Nutrient-Rich: Bell peppers are low in calories but packed with important vitamins and minerals.

Zucchini Noodles with Pesto

Preparation Time: 15 minutes

Cooking Time: 5 minutes

Servings: 2

Ingredients:

- 2 medium zucchinis
- Homemade or store-bought pesto sauce (low-fat)
- Cherry tomatoes, split
- Pine nuts (extra)
- Fresh basil leaves for garnish
- Salt and pepper to taste

Instructions:

- Use a spiralizer or veggie knife to make zucchini noodles.

- In a pan over medium heat, lightly sauté the zucchini noodles for about 3-5 minutes until they soften slightly.

- Toss the zucchini noodles with pesto sauce until evenly coated.

- Add cherry tomatoes and pine nuts (if using). Stir gently to mix.

- Season with salt and pepper.

- Garnish with fresh basil leaves before serving.

Nutritional Value (Per Serving)::

Calories: Approximately 120, Protein: 3g, Carbohydrates: 10g, Fat: 8g, Fiber: 3g

Health Benefits and Nutritional Insights:

1. Low-Calorie Alternative: Zucchini noodles offer a low-calorie alternative for standard pasta.

2. Rich in Vitamins: Zucchinis are rich in vitamins and minerals, adding to a nutrient-dense meal.

Black Bean and Corn Salad

Preparation Time: 15 minutes

Servings: 4-6

Ingredients:

- Black beans, washed and drained, in one can (15 ounces).

- 1 cup corn kernels (fresh or warmed if frozen)

- 1 red bell pepper, diced

- 1/2 red onion, roughly chopped

- 1 jalapeño, sliced and diced (optional for heat)
- Fresh cilantro, chopped
- Juice of 2 limes
- 2 tablespoons olive oil
- Salt and pepper to taste
- Avocado (extra for decoration)

Instructions:

- In a big mixing bowl, add black beans, corn, diced red bell pepper, chopped red onion, diced jalapeño (if using), and fresh cilantro.
- In a separate small bowl, mix together lime juice, olive oil, salt, and pepper.
- Pour the dressing over the bean mixture and toss until well mixed.
- Taste and adjust spice if needed.

- Garnish with chopped avocado (if wanted) before serving.

Nutritional Value (Per Serving)::

Calories: Approximately 150, Protein: 6g, Carbohydrates: 23g, Fat: 5g, Fiber: 6g

Health Benefits and Nutritional Insights:

1. Rich in Fiber and Protein: Black beans are a great source of fiber and protein.
2. Vitamin-Packed: This salad is filled with vitamins from different veggies, supporting general health.

Cauliflower Fried Rice

Preparation Time: 15 minutes

Cooking Time: 10 minutes

Servings: 4

Ingredients:

- 1 medium head cauliflower, chopped or crushed into rice-like texture
- 1 cup mixed veggies (peas, carrots, corn)
- 2 cloves garlic, minced
- 1 small onion, roughly chopped
- 2 tablespoons low-sodium soy sauce or tamari
- 1 tablespoon sesame oil
- 2 green onions, chopped (for garnish)
- Sesame seeds (optional, for garnish)
- Salt and pepper to taste

Instructions:

- In a big pan or wok, heat sesame oil over medium heat.
- Add crushed garlic and chopped onion, sauté until fragrant and onions are yellow.
- Add the mixed veggies and cook until they start to soften.
- Add the cauliflower rice and stir-fry for 5-7 minutes until it gets the required softness.
- Pour soy sauce over the ingredients and stir until evenly mixed. Season with salt and pepper.
- Before serving, garnish with sesame seeds and finely chopped green onions.

Nutritional Value (Per Serving)::

Calories: Approximately 100, Protein: 5g, Carbohydrates: 15g, Fat: 3g, Fiber: 5g

Health Benefits and Nutritional Insights:

1. Low-Carb Alternative: Cauliflower rice is a low-carb alternative for regular rice.
2. Vitamin-Rich: This food is packed with veggies, giving different vitamins and minerals.

Chickpea and Spinach Curry

Preparation Time: 10 minutes

Cooking Time: 20 minutes

Servings: 4

Ingredients:

- 2 cans (15 ounces each) chickpeas, drained and washed
- 1 onion, roughly chopped
- 3 cloves garlic, minced
- 1 teaspoon chopped ginger
- 1 can (14 ounces) diced tomatoes
- 2 cups fresh spinach leaves
- 1 can (14 ounces) coconut milk
- 2 tablespoons curry powder
- 1 teaspoon ground turmeric
- 1 teaspoon crushed cumin
- 1 tablespoon olive oil
- Salt and pepper to taste
- Fresh parsley for garnish

Instructions:

- In a large pan, warm up the olive oil over medium heat. Add chopped onion and sauté until translucent.
- Add chopped garlic and grated ginger, cook for another minute until fragrant.

- Stir in curry powder, ground turmeric, and ground cumin, cook for 1-2 minutes.
- Add diced tomatoes, chickpeas, and coconut milk. Simmer for 10 minutes.
- Fold in fresh spinach and cook for an extra 5 minutes until the spinach wilts.
- Season with salt and pepper to taste.
- Garnish with fresh cilantro before serving.

Nutritional Value (Per Serving)::

Calories: Approximately 160, Protein: 6g, Carbohydrates: 18g, Fat: 8g, Fiber: 6g

Health Benefits and Nutritional Insights:

1. Rich in Protein and Fiber: Chickpeas provide protein and fiber, helping in satisfaction and digestion.
2. Vitamin-Packed: Spinach is rich in vitamins and minerals, adding to a nutrient-dense meal.

Stuffed Portobello Mushrooms

Preparation Time: 15 minutes

Cooking Time: 20 minutes

Servings: 4

Ingredients:

- 4 big Portobello mushrooms, tips removed
- 1 cup spinach, chopped
- 1/2 cup cherry tomatoes, diced
- 1/2 cup red bell pepper, diced

- 1/4 cup red onion, finely chopped
- 2 cloves garlic, minced
- 1/2 cup breadcrumbs (whole wheat for healthy choice)
- 1/4 cup grated Parmesan cheese (optional or use a veggie replacement)
- 2 tablespoons olive oil
- Fresh basil leaves for garnish
- Salt and pepper to taste

Instructions:

- Preheat the oven to 375°F (190°C). The Portobello mushrooms should be put on a baking pan.
- Warm up some olive oil in a pan over medium heat. Add chopped garlic and sauté until fragrant.
- Add chopped spinach, cherry tomatoes, red bell pepper, and red onion. Allow vegetables to soften for 3–4 minutes.
- Stir in breadcrumbs and chopped Parmesan cheese (if using). Cook for an extra minute.
- Stuff each Portobello mushroom cap with the veggie mixture.
- Bake for 15-20 minutes until mushrooms are soft and filling is golden brown.
- Garnish with fresh basil leaves before serving.

Nutritional Value (Per Serving)::

Calories: Approximately 130, Protein: 5g, Carbohydrates: 14g, Fat: 7g, Fiber: 4g

Health Benefits and Nutritional Insights:

1. Low-Calorie and Fiber-Rich:
   Portobello mushrooms are low
   in calories and high in fiber,
   helping in digestion.
2. Nutrient-Dense: This food is
   packed with different veggies,
   giving important vitamins and
   minerals.

Eggplant and Tomato Bake

Preparation Time: 20 minutes

Cooking Time: 30 minutes

Servings: 4

Ingredients:

- 2 medium eggplants, sliced
  into rounds
- 4 tomatoes, sliced
- 2 cloves garlic, minced
- 1/4 cup fresh basil leaves,
  chopped
- 1/4 cup fresh parsley, chopped
- 1/4 cup grated Parmesan
  cheese (optional or use a
  veggie replacement)
- 2 tablespoons olive oil
- Salt and pepper to taste

Instructions:

- Preheat the oven to 375°F
  (190°C). Grease a baking dish
  with olive oil.
- Layer the eggplant rounds at
  the bottom of the baking dish.
- Top the eggplant with
  chopped garlic, cut tomatoes,
  fresh basil, and parsley.
- Drizzle olive oil over the top
  and season with salt and
  pepper.
- Bake the dish for 20 minutes
  with the foil covering it.

- Uncover, sprinkle grated Parmesan cheese (if using), and bake for an additional 10 minutes until eggplant is soft and cheese is golden.

Nutritional Value (Per Serving)::

Calories: Approximately 120, Protein: 4g, Carbohydrates: 16g, Fat: 6g, Fiber: 8g

Health Benefits and Nutritional Insights:

1. Low-Calorie and Nutrient-Rich: Eggplants are low in calories and provide important nutrients like fiber and vitamins.
2. Vitamin-Packed: Tomatoes are rich in vitamins, especially vitamin C, supporting general health.

Veggie Stir-Fry with Tofu

Preparation Time: 15 minutes

Cooking Time: 15 minutes

Servings: 4

Ingredients:

- 1 block firm tofu, pressed and cubed
- 2 cups mixed veggies (broccoli, bell peppers, snap peas, carrots)
- 1 onion, sliced
- 3 cloves garlic, minced
- 1 tablespoon ginger, grated
- 3 tablespoons low-sodium soy sauce or tamari
- 1 tablespoon rice vinegar
- 1 tablespoon sesame oil
- 1 tablespoon cornstarch (two tablespoons water combined)

- 2 tablespoons chopped green onions for garnish
- Sesame seeds for decoration (optional)
- Salt and pepper to taste

Instructions:

- Heat sesame oil in a big pan or wok over medium-high heat.
- Add cubed tofu and stir-fry until golden brown on all sides. Take out the tofu and put it aside.
- In the same pan, add sliced onion, minced garlic, and chopped ginger. Sauté for a minute until fragrant.
- Add mixed veggies to the pan and stir-fry for 3-4 minutes until they start to soften.
- In a small bowl, mix soy sauce, rice vinegar, and the cornstarch-water mixture. Pour over the veggies.
- Add the cooked tofu back into the pan and toss everything together until the sauce thickens.
- Season with salt and pepper to taste.
- Before serving, garnish with sesame seeds and finely chopped green onions.

Nutritional Value (Per Serving)::

Calories: Approximately 150, Protein: 10g, Carbohydrates: 12g, Fat: 8g, Fiber: 4g

Health Benefits and Nutritional Insights:

1. High-energy: Tofu offers a good amount of plant-based energy.

2. Vitamin-Rich: Mixed veggies offer different vitamins and minerals, improving the nutritional balance.

Lentil and Vegetable Soup

Preparation Time: 15 minutes

Cooking Time: 30 minutes

Servings: 6

Ingredients:

- 1 cup dried lentils, rinsed
- 6 cups vegetable broth
- 2 carrots, diced
- 2 celery stalks, diced
- 1 onion, chopped
- 3 cloves garlic, minced
- 1 can (14 ounces) diced tomatoes
- 1 teaspoon dried thyme
- 1 teaspoon dried oregano
- 1 bay leaf
- 2 tablespoons olive oil
- Fresh parsley for garnish
- Salt and pepper to taste

Instructions:

- In a big saucepan, warm the olive oil over medium heat. Add chopped onion, sliced garlic, cut carrots, and celery. Sauté until veggies begin to soften.
- Add washed lentils, diced tomatoes, veggie broth, dried thyme, dried oregano, and bay leaf to the pot. Bring to a boil.
- Reduce heat to low, cover, and simmer for 25-30 minutes until lentils are soft.
- Remove the bay leaf and season with salt and pepper to taste.

- Garnish with fresh parsley before serving.

Nutritional Value (Per Serving)::

Calories: Approximately 160, Protein: 9g, Carbohydrates: 24g, Fat: 4g, Fiber: 8g

Health Benefits and Nutritional Insights:

1. Rich in Protein and Fiber: Lentils provide both protein and fiber, helping in digestion and satisfaction.
2. Vitamin-Packed: This soup is packed with veggies, giving different vitamins and minerals.

Quinoa and Black Bean Salad

Preparation Time: 20 minutes

Servings: 4

Ingredients:

- 1 cup quinoa, rinsed
- Washing and draining one can (15 ounces) of black beans
- 1 red bell pepper, diced
- 1/2 cup corn kernels (fresh, canned, or warmed if frozen)
- 1/4 cup red onion, finely chopped
- 1/4 cup fresh cilantro, chopped
- Juice of 2 limes
- 2 tablespoons olive oil
- 1 teaspoon crushed cumin
- Salt and pepper to taste
- Avocado slices for decoration (optional)

Instructions:

- Cook quinoa according to package directions. Once cooked, fluff with a fork and let it cool.
- In a large mixing bowl, add cooked quinoa, black beans, diced red bell pepper, corn kernels, chopped red onion, and fresh cilantro.
- In a separate small bowl, mix together lime juice, olive oil, ground cumin, salt, and pepper.
- Pour the dressing over the rice mixture and toss until well mixed.
- Taste and adjust spice if needed.
- Garnish with avocado slices before serving (if wanted).

Nutritional Value (Per Serving)::

Calories: Approximately 220, Protein: 9g, Carbohydrates: 33g, Fat: 7g, Fiber: 8g,

Health Benefits and Nutritional Insights:

1. Protein and Fiber-Rich: Both quinoa and black beans provide a good amount of protein and fiber.
2. Vitamin-Packed: This salad is filled with veggies, giving different vitamins and minerals.

Chickpea Avocado Salad

Preparation Time: 15 minutes

Servings: 4

Ingredients:

- 2 cans (15 ounces each) chickpeas, drained and washed
- 2 avocados, diced
- 1 cucumber, diced
- 1/4 cup red onion, finely chopped
- 1/4 cup fresh parsley, chopped
- Juice of 1 lemon
- 2 tablespoons olive oil
- 1 teaspoon cumin
- Salt and pepper to taste

Instructions:

- In a big mixing bowl, add beans, diced avocados, diced cucumber, chopped red onion, and fresh parsley.
- In a separate small bowl, mix together lemon juice, olive oil, cumin, salt, and pepper.
- Pour the dressing over the salad ingredients and toss until well mixed.
- Taste and adjust spice if needed.

Nutritional Value (Per Serving)::

Calories: Approximately 280, Protein: 9g, Carbohydrates: 28g, Fat: 15g, Fiber: 10g

Health Benefits and Nutritional Insights:

1. Protein and Healthy Fats: This salad mixes beans and avocado, giving a good amount of protein and healthy fats.
2. Nutrient-Rich: It's packed with fiber and different nutrients from the products used.

Mediterranean Quinoa Salad

Preparation Time: 20 minutes

Servings: 4

Ingredients:

- 1 cup quinoa, rinsed
- 1 cup cherry tomatoes, sliced
- 1 cucumber, diced
- 1/2 cup Kalamata olives, chopped and sliced
- 1/4 cup red onion, finely chopped
- 1/4 cup fresh parsley, chopped
- 1/4 cup fresh mint leaves, chopped
- Juice of 1 lemon
- 3 tablespoons extra-virgin olive oil
- 1 teaspoon dried oregano
- Salt and pepper to taste
- Crumbled feta cheese (extra)

Instructions:

- Cook quinoa according to package directions. Once cooked, fluff with a fork and let it cool.
- In a large mixing bowl, add cooked quinoa, split cherry tomatoes, diced cucumber, sliced Kalamata olives, chopped red onion, fresh parsley, and fresh mint leaves.
- In a separate small bowl, mix together lemon juice, extra-virgin olive oil, dried oregano, salt, and pepper.
- Pour the dressing over the salad ingredients and toss until well mixed.
- Top with chopped feta cheese if wanted before serving.

Nutritional Value (Per Serving)::

Calories: Approximately 240,

Protein: 6g, Carbohydrates: 28g,

Fat: 12g, Fiber: 5g

Health Benefits and Nutritional Insights:

1. Protein and Nutrient-Dense: Quinoa offers protein and different nutrients, while the veggies add vitamins and minerals.
2. Mediterranean tastes: Incorporating olives and olive oil offers healthy fats and unique Mediterranean tastes.

<u>Vegan Chickpea Curry</u>

Preparation Time: 15 minutes

Cooking Time: 25 minutes

Servings: 4

Ingredients:

- 2 cans (15 ounces each) chickpeas, drained and washed
- 1 onion, roughly chopped
- 3 cloves garlic, minced
- 1 tablespoon fresh ginger, chopped
- 1 can (14 ounces) diced tomatoes
- 1 can (14 ounces) coconut milk
- 2 cups spinach leaves
- 2 tablespoons curry powder
- 1 teaspoon ground turmeric
- 1 teaspoon crushed cumin
- 1 tablespoon coconut oil
- Salt and pepper to taste
- Fresh parsley for garnish

Instructions:

- Heat coconut oil in a big pan over medium heat. Add chopped onion and sauté until translucent.
- Add chopped garlic and grated ginger, cook for another minute until fragrant.
- Stir in curry powder, ground turmeric, and ground cumin, cook for 1-2 minutes.
- Add diced tomatoes, chickpeas, and coconut milk. Simmer for 10 minutes.
- Fold in fresh spinach and cook for an extra 5 minutes until the spinach wilts.
- Season with salt and pepper to taste.
- Garnish with fresh cilantro before serving.

Nutritional Value (Per Serving)::

Calories: Approximately 260, Protein: 10g, Carbohydrates: 30g, Fat: 12g, Fiber: 9g

Health Benefits and Nutritional Insights:

1. Plant-Based Protein: Chickpeas are a great source of protein, making this curry satisfying and healthy.
2. Vitamin-Rich: Spinach adds vitamins and minerals, improving the dish's nutritional profile.

Vegan Lentil Shepherd's Pie

Preparation Time: 25 minutes

Cooking Time: 40 minutes

Servings: 6

Ingredients

For the Filling:

- 1 cup dry green or brown lentils, cleaned
- 3 cups vegetable broth
- 1 onion, diced
- 2 carrots, diced
- 2 cloves garlic, minced
- 1 cup frozen peas
- 1 tablespoon tomato sauce
- 1 teaspoon dried thyme
- 1 teaspoon dried rosemary
- Salt and pepper to taste
- 2 tablespoons olive oil

For the Mashed Potato Topping:

- 4 large potatoes, peeled and cubed
- 1/4 cup plain almond milk or any plant-based milk
- 2 tablespoons vegan butter
- Salt and pepper to taste

Instructions:

For the Filling:

- In a pot, mix beans and veggie broth. Bring to a boil, then reduce heat and cook for 20-25 minutes until lentils are soft and the liquid is absorbed.
- In a different pan, heat olive oil over medium heat. Add diced onion, carrots, and garlic. Sauté until softened.
- Add cooked lentils, frozen peas, tomato paste, dried thyme, dried rosemary, salt, and pepper to the onion and carrot blend. Cook for an extra 5 minutes. Set aside.

For the Mashed Potato Topping:

- Boil the cubed potatoes in a pot of salted water until soft. Drain well.

- Mash the potatoes while they're still warm. Stir in vegan butter, almond milk, salt, and pepper. Mix until smooth and creamy.
- Assembling the Shepherd's Pie:
- Preheat the oven to 375°F (190°C).
- Transfer the bean and veggie mixture into a baking dish.
- Spread the mashed potatoes over the lentil mixture evenly.
- Bake for 20-25 minutes or until the top is golden brown.
- Serve hot.

Nutritional Value (Per Serving)::

Calories: Approximately 320, Protein: 13g, Carbohydrates: 52g, Fat: 7g, Fiber: 11g

Health Benefits and Nutritional Insights:

1. High in Fiber and Protein: Lentils provide fiber and protein, adding to a healthy meal.
2. Vitamins and Minerals: This food is rich in vitamins from veggies and beans.

Chickpea Salad Sandwich Filling

Preparation Time: 15 minutes

Servings: 4-6

Ingredients:

- 2 cans (15 ounces each) chickpeas, drained and washed
- 1/2 cup celery, finely chopped
- 1/4 cup red onion, finely chopped

- 1/4 cup fresh parsley, finely chopped
- 1/4 cup vegan mayonnaise
- 1 tablespoon Dijon mustard
- 1 tablespoon lemon juice
- 1/2 teaspoon garlic powder
- Salt and pepper to taste
- Lettuce leaves
- Sliced bread or sandwich rolls

Instructions:

- In a large bowl, mash the chickpeas using a fork or potato masher until chunky.
- Add chopped celery, red onion, and fresh parsley to the cooked chickpeas.
- In a separate small bowl, mix together vegan mayonnaise, Dijon mustard, lemon juice, garlic powder, salt, and pepper.
- Pour the sauce over the chickpea mixture and stir until well mixed.
- Taste and adjust spice if needed.
- Serve the chickpea salad on cut bread or sandwich rolls with green leaves.

Nutritional Value (Per Serving)::

Calories: Approximately 230, Protein: 9g, Carbohydrates: 28g, Fat: 8g, Fiber: 8g

Health Benefits and Nutritional Insights:

1. energy-Rich: Chickpeas provide a good amount of plant-based energy.
2. Fiber and Flavor: The veggies and herbs add fiber and improve the general taste.

Vegan Black Bean Burger

Preparation Time: 20 minutes

Cooking Time: 10 minutes

Servings: 4

Ingredients:

- 2 cans (15 ounces each) black beans, drained and washed
- Half a cup of whole wheat or gluten-free bread crumbs
- 1/4 cup red onion, finely chopped
- 1/4 cup bell peppers (any color), finely chopped
- 2 cloves garlic, minced
- 2 cups fresh cilantro, chopped
- 1 tablespoon ground cumin
- 1 teaspoon paprika
- Salt and pepper to taste
- Olive oil for cooking
- Burger buns
- Toppings of choice (lettuce, tomato, avocado, etc.)

Instructions:

- In a mixing bowl, mash half of the black beans until a paste forms. Add the leftover beans and lightly mash, leaving some whole beans for structure.
- Add bread crumbs, chopped red onion, chopped bell peppers, minced garlic, fresh cilantro, ground cumin, paprika, salt, and pepper to the cooked beans. Mix until well mixed.
- Divide the mixture into 4 equal pieces and make them into burger patties.

- The olive oil should be warmed in a pan over medium heat. Cook the patties for 4-5 minutes on each side or until they grow a crispy top.
- Serve the black bean burgers on burger buns with your pick of toppings.

Nutritional Value (Per Serving, without bun and toppings):

Calories: Approximately 230, Protein: 13g, Carbohydrates: 38g, Fat: 2g, Fiber: 13g

Health Benefits and Nutritional Insights:

1. Protein and Fiber-Rich: Black beans provide a good amount of protein and fiber.
2. Low in Fat: This veggie burger is low in fat compared to regular meat-based burgers.

Preparation Time: 15 minutes

Servings: 4 wraps

Ingredients:

- 1 can (15 ounces) chickpeas, drained and washed
- 1/4 cup vegan mayonnaise
- 2 tablespoons lemon juice
- 1/4 cup red onion, finely chopped
- 1/4 cup celery, roughly chopped
- 2 cups fresh parsley, chopped
- Salt and pepper to taste
- 4 big whole grain wraps
- Lettuce greens or spinach for building
- Sliced tomatoes and avocado for filling

Instructions:

- In a large bowl, mash the chickpeas using a fork or potato masher until partly mashed.
- Add vegan mayonnaise, lemon juice, red onion, celery, and fresh parsley to the mashed chickpeas. Mix well to mix.
- Toss to season with salt and pepper to taste.
- Lay out the whole grain wraps on a clean surface. Place a few lettuce leaves or spinach in the middle of each wrap.
- Divide the chickpea salad evenly among the wraps, spreading it over the lettuce leaves or spinach.
- Add pieces of tomato and avocado on top of the chickpea salad.
- Fold the sides of the wraps towards the center, then roll them tightly.
- Once each wrap is diagonally cut in half, serve.

Nutritional Value (Per Serving, 1 Wrap):

Calories: Approximately 280, Protein: 10g, Carbohydrates: 40g, Fat: 9g, Fiber: 8g

Health Benefits and Nutritional Insights:

1. Protein and Fiber: Chickpeas provide a good amount of protein and fiber, boosting fullness and helping in digestion.
2. Vitamins and Minerals: Ingredients like red onion, celery, and parsley offer

different vitamins and minerals.

Vegan Eggplant and Chickpea Curry

Preparation Time: 20 minutes

Cooking Time: 25 minutes

Servings: 4

Ingredients:

- 1 big eggplant, diced
- 1 can (15 ounces) chickpeas, drained and washed
- 1 onion, roughly chopped
- 3 cloves garlic, minced
- 1-inch piece of ginger, grated
- 1 can (14 ounces) diced tomatoes
- 1 can (14 ounces) coconut milk
- 2 tablespoons curry powder
- 1 teaspoon crushed cumin
- 1 teaspoon chopped coriander
- 1 teaspoon turmeric
- 1 tablespoon olive oil
- Salt and pepper to taste
- Fresh parsley for garnish

Instructions:

- Heat olive oil in a big pan or pot over medium heat. Add chopped onion and sauté until translucent.
- Add chopped garlic and grated ginger, cook for another minute until fragrant.
- Stir in curry powder, ground cumin, ground coriander, and turmeric, cooking for 1-2 minutes.
- Add diced eggplant and beans to the pan, turning to coat with the spices.

- Pour in the chopped tomatoes and coconut milk. Simmer for 15-20 minutes until the eggplant is soft and the curry thickens.
- Season with salt and pepper to taste.
- Garnish with fresh cilantro before serving.

Nutritional Value (Per Serving)::

Calories: Approximately 260, Protein: 9g, Carbohydrates: 28g, Fat: 13g, Fiber: 11g

Health Benefits and Nutritional Insights:

1. High in Fiber and Flavorful: This curry mixes eggplant and chickpeas, giving fiber and a burst of flavors from the spices.

2. Vegan Protein: Chickpeas offer a good amount of plant-based protein.

Asparagus and Cherry Tomato Pasta

Preparation Time: 20 minutes

Cooking Time: 15 minutes

Servings: 4

Ingredients:

- Eight ounces of your favorite pasta, or whole wheat spaghetti
- 1 bunch asparagus, trimmed and cut into 1-inch pieces
- 1 pint cherry tomatoes, split
- 3 cloves garlic, minced
- 1/4 cup fresh basil leaves, chopped

- 2 tablespoons olive oil

- Juice of 1 lemon

- Zest of 1 lemon

- Salt and pepper to taste

- Grated Parmesan cheese or healthy yeast for serving (alternative)

Instructions:

- Cook the pasta according to package guidelines in a pot of salted boiling water until al dente. Drain and set away, saving about 1/2 cup of pasta water.

- While the pasta is cooking, heat olive oil in a large pan over medium heat. Cook the chopped garlic for one minute, or until it becomes aromatic.

- Add the asparagus pieces to the pan and sauté for 3-4 minutes until they start to become soft.

- Add the split cherry tomatoes to the pan and continue to cook for another 2-3 minutes until they start to soften.

- Toss in the cooked pasta, lemon juice, lemon zest, and chopped basil. Toss everything together until well mixed. If needed, add a bit of leftover pasta water to loosen the pasta.

- Season with salt and pepper to taste.

- Serve the Asparagus and Cherry Tomato Pasta with added grated Parmesan cheese or healthy yeast.

Nutritional Value (Approximate per Serving):

Calories: Approximately 300,
Protein: 9g, Carbohydrates: 50g,
Fat: 8g, Fiber: 8g

Health Benefits and Nutritional Insights:

1. Asparagus Nutrition: Asparagus is rich in folate, vitamins A, C, and K, and offers a good bit of fiber.
2. Cherry Tomatoes: Cherry tomatoes offer vitamins like lycopene and are low in calories but high in nutrients.

Roasted Brussels Sprouts with Balsamic Glaze

Preparation Time: 10 minutes

Cooking Time: 25 minutes

Servings: 4

Ingredients:

- 1 pound Brussels sprouts, cut and split
- 2 tablespoons olive oil
- Salt and pepper to taste
- 2 tablespoons balsamic sauce (store-bought or homemade)
- Optional: Grated Parmesan cheese or healthy yeast for serving

Instructions:

- Adjust the oven temperature to 400°F (200°C) and place parchment paper on a baking pan.
- In a mixing bowl, toss the split Brussels sprouts with olive oil, salt, and pepper until thoroughly covered.

- Spread the Brussels sprouts in a single line on the prepared baking sheet.
- Roast in the warm oven for 20-25 minutes, stirring halfway through, until the Brussels sprouts are golden brown and soft when poked with a fork.
- Remove the roasted Brussels sprouts from the oven and transfer them to a serving dish.
- Drizzle the balsamic sauce over the roasted Brussels sprouts and toss gently to coat evenly.
- Serve the Roasted Brussels Sprouts with a sprinkle of chopped Parmesan cheese or nutritional yeast if preferred.

Nutritional Value (Approximate per Serving):

Calories: Approximately 100, Protein: 3g, Carbohydrates: 10g, Fat: 6g, Fiber: 4g

Health Benefits and Nutritional Insights:

1. Brussels Sprouts Nutrition: Brussels sprouts are rich in vitamins K and C, calcium, and antioxidants.
2. Balsamic Glaze: The balsamic glaze adds a tangy sweetness and is a lower-calorie option to heavy sauces.

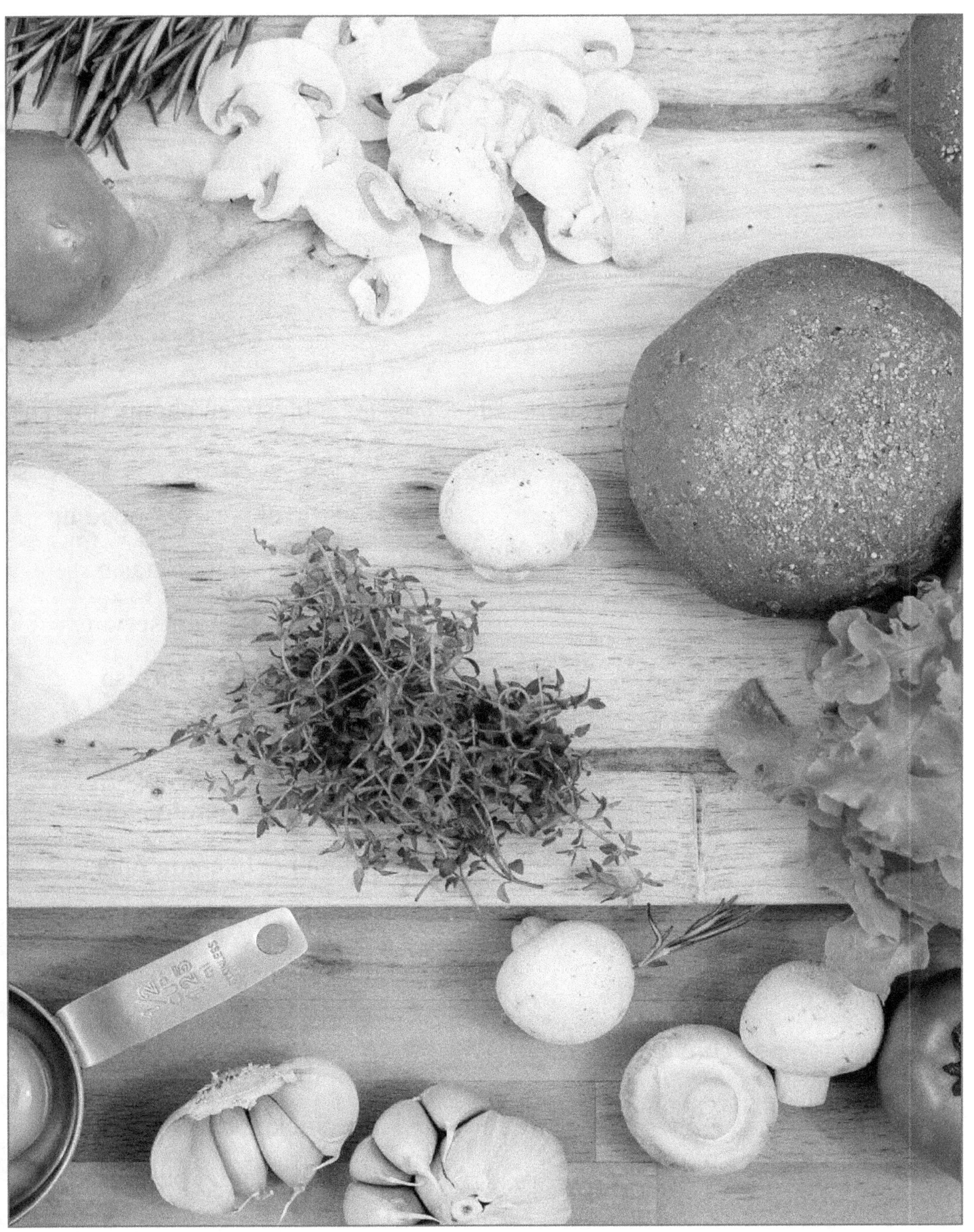

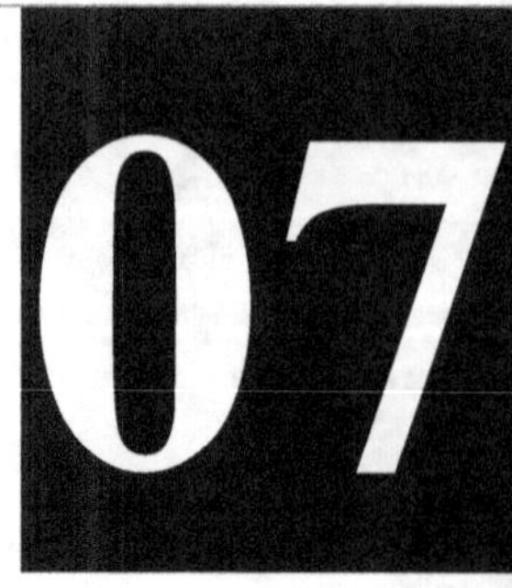

Lemon herb chicken on the grill

Preparation Time: 10 minutes (plus time to marinate).

Cooking Time: 15 minutes.

Servings: 4

Ingredients:

- 4 chicken breasts without bones or skin
- 2 tablespoons olive oil
- Two lemons' zest and juice
- 2 tablespoons of chopped fresh rosemary
- 1/2 tablespoon chopped fresh thyme
- 3 garlic cloves, chopped up
- Salt and pepper to taste
- Lemon pieces for serving
- Fresh herbs for garnish

Instructions:

- In a bowl, mix olive oil, lemon peel, lemon juice, chopped rosemary, chopped thyme, sliced garlic, salt, and pepper to make the marinade.
- Seal the plastic bag or place the chicken breasts in a shallow plate. Pour the

marinade over the chicken, ensuring it's evenly coated. Let it marinate for at least half an hour, or better still, all night.

- Preheat the grill to medium-high heat.
- Grill the chicken for 6-8 minutes per side or until it hits an internal temperature of 165°F (74°C) and has grill marks.
- Serve with lemon wedges and top with fresh herbs.

Nutritional Values (per serving):

Calories: Approximately 200, Protein: 25g, Fat: 9g, Carbohydrates: 2g, Fiber: 1g

Health Benefits:

1. Chicken is a lean source of energy.

2. Olive oil gives heart-healthy monounsaturated fats.

3. Lemon, oregano, and thyme add taste without extra calories.

4. Garlic adds possible health benefits.

Baked Garlic Parmesan Chicken Tenders

Preparation Time: 15 minutes

Cooking Time: 20 minutes

Servings: 4

Ingredients:

- 1 lb chicken tenders
- 1 cup whole wheat breadcrumbs
- 1/2 cup grated Parmesan cheese

- 2 tsp garlic powder
- 1 teaspoon onion powder
- 1 teaspoon dried oregano
- Salt and pepper to taste
- 2 large eggs, beaten
- Cooking spray
- Fresh parsley for garnish
- Marinara sauce for dipping (optional)

Instructions:

- Preheat the oven to 400°F (200°C).
- In a bowl, mix whole wheat breadcrumbs, chopped Parmesan cheese, garlic powder, onion powder, dried oregano, salt, and pepper.
- Dip each chicken tender into the beaten eggs, then coat it with the breadcrumb mixture, pressing gently to attach.
- Place the coated chicken tenders on a baking sheet lined with parchment paper and lightly cover with cooking spray.
- Bake the chicken for 18 to 20 minutes, or until it is cooked through and has a golden brown color.
- Garnish with fresh herbs and serve with marinara sauce for dipping if preferred.

Nutritional Values (per serving):

Calories: Approximately 250, Protein: 30g, Fat: 8g, Carbohydrates: 15g Fiber: 3g

Health Benefits:

1. Chicken strips provide a lean source of energy.
2. Whole wheat breadcrumbs add fiber and protein.

3. Parmesan cheese adds calcium and taste.

4. Garlic and thyme add delicious notes without extra calories.

Slow Cooker Salsa Chicken

Preparation Time: 10 minutes

Cooking Time: 4-6 hours (slow pot)

Servings: 4

Ingredients:

- 4 chicken breasts without bones or skin
- 1 cup salsa (choose your desired heat level)
- 1 teaspoon crushed cumin
- 1 teaspoon pepper spice
- 1 teaspoon garlic powder
- Salt and pepper to taste
- Fresh parsley for decoration (optional)
- Lime pieces for serving

Instructions:

- Place chicken breasts in the slow cooker.
- In a bowl, mix salsa, ground cumin, chili powder, garlic powder, salt, and pepper.
- Pour the salsa sauce over the chicken, ensuring it's well-coated.
- Cook on low for 4-6 hours or until the chicken is soft and easily shreds with a fork.
- Shred the chicken straight in the slow cooker and mix it with the salsa.

- Fresh cilantro is used as a garnish and served with lime wedges.

Nutritional Values (per serving):

Calories: Approximately 180
Protein: 25g, Fat: 3g,
Carbohydrates: 10g, Fiber: 2g

Health Benefits:

1. Chicken is a lean source of energy.
2. Salsa adds taste without extra calories and offers vitamins from veggies.
3. Cumin and chili powder add a warm and spicy taste.
4. This recipe is low in fat and can be customized based on spice preferences.

Sheet Pan Balsamic Chicken and Vegetables

Preparation Time: 15 minutes

Cooking Time: 25 minutes

Servings: 4

Ingredients:

- 4 chicken breasts without bones or skin
- 1 cup cherry tomatoes, halved
- 1 bell pepper, sliced
- 1 zucchini, chopped/
- 1 red onion, sliced
- 3 tablespoons balsamic vinegar
- 2 tablespoons olive oil
- 2 teaspoons Dijon mustard
- 1 teaspoon dried rosemary
- Salt and pepper to taste
- Fresh basil for garnish

Instructions:

- Preheat the oven to 400°F (200°C).
- Arrange the chicken breasts on a parchment paper-lined baking pan.
- In a bowl, whisk together balsamic vinegar, olive oil, Dijon mustard, dried rosemary, salt, and pepper.
- Toss cherry tomatoes, bell pepper, zucchini, and red onion in the balsamic mixture.
- On the baking sheet, arrange the veggies around the chicken.
- Bake for 20 to 25 minutes, or until the vegetables are tender and the chicken is well cooked.
- Garnish with fresh basil before presenting.

Nutritional Values (per serving):

Calories: Approximately 250,

Protein: 30g, Fat: 10g,

Carbohydrates: 10g, Fiber: 3g

Health Benefits:

1. Chicken gives lean energy.
2. A variety of vitamins, minerals, and fiber may be found in vegetables.
3. Balsamic vinegar and olive oil add taste without extra calories.
4. This recipe is low in carbs and ideal for a healthy meal
5.

Instant Pot Shredded Chicken Tacos

Preparation Time: 10 minutes

Cooking Time: 20 minutes (plus time for the Instant Pot to pressurize)

Servings: 4

Ingredients:

- lbs boneless, skinless chicken breasts
- 1 cup chicken broth
- 1 cup salsa
- 1 tablespoon ground cumin
- 1 tablespoon pepper spice
- 1 teaspoon garlic powder
- 1 teaspoon onion powder
- 1/2 teaspoon smoked pepper
- Salt and pepper to taste
- Corn or whole wheat tortillas
- Toppings: Shredded lettuce, diced tomatoes, shredded cheese, Greek yogurt or low-fat sour cream, lime wedges, fresh cilantro

Instructions:

- Place chicken breasts in the Instant Pot.
- In a bowl, mix chicken broth, salsa, ground cumin, chili powder, garlic powder, onion powder, smoked paprika, salt, and pepper.
- Pour the liquid over the chicken in the Instant Pot.
- Close the Instant Pot lid, set to "Sealing," and cook on high pressure for 15 minutes.
- Allow for natural pressure release for 5 minutes, then physically release the leftover pressure.
- Shred the chicken using two forks straight in the Instant Pot.
- Serve the chopped chicken in tacos with chosen toppings.

Nutritional Values (per serving):

Calories: Approximately 250

Protein: 30g, Fat: 5g,

Carbohydrates: 20g, Fiber: 3g

Health Benefits:

1) Chicken offers a lean amount of energy.
2) Salsa gives taste without extra calories.
3) Spices like cumin, pepper powder, and garlic powder add taste and possible health benefits.
4) Toppings like lettuce, peppers, and Greek yogurt add freshness and additional benefits.

Herb-Roasted Turkey Breast

Herb-Roasted Turkey Breast

Preparation Time: 15 minutes

Cooking Time: 1.5 to 2 hours

Servings: 6

Ingredients:

- 3 lbs bone-in turkey breast, skin-on
- 2 tablespoons olive oil
- 2 teaspoons dried thyme
- 2 teaspoons dried rosemary
- 2 teaspoons dried sage
- 1 teaspoon garlic powder
- 1 teaspoon onion powder
- Salt and pepper to taste
- 1 cup chicken broth (for cooking)

Instructions:

- Preheat the oven to 325°F (163°C).
- In a small bowl, mix olive oil, dried thyme, dried rosemary,

dried sage, garlic powder, onion powder, salt, and pepper to make the herb rub.

- Pat the turkey breast dry with paper towels. Rub the herb mixture all over and under the skin of the turkey.
- Place the turkey breast on a rack in a baking pan, skin side up.
- Fill the roasting pan's bottom with chicken broth.
- Roast the turkey for 1.5 to 2 hours or until the internal temperature reaches 165°F (74°C), basting with pan juices every 30 minutes.
- Before slicing, let the turkey 15 minutes to rest.

Nutritional Values (per serving):

Calories: Approximately 200, Protein: 25g, Fat: 9g, Carbohydrates: 0g, Fiber: 0g

Health Benefits:

2. Turkey breast is a lean source of energy.
3. Olive oil gives heart-healthy monounsaturated fats.
4. Herbs like thyme, rosemary, and sage add taste without extra calories.
5. This recipe is low in carbs, making it ideal for a healthy meal.

Lemon Pepper Chicken Skewers

Preparation Time: 20 minutes (including marination)

Cooking Time: 10-12 minutes

Servings: 4

Ingredients:

- lbs boneless, skinless chicken breasts, cut into cubes
- Two lemons' zest and juice
- 2 tablespoons olive oil
- 1 teaspoon black pepper
- 1 teaspoon dried oregano
- 1 teaspoon garlic powder
- Salt to taste
- Wooden or metal skewers, wet if wooden
- Lemon pieces for serving
- Fresh parsley for garnish

Instructions:

- In a bowl, mix olive oil, lemon zest, lemon juice, black pepper, dried oregano, garlic powder, and salt to make the marinade.
- Add the chicken bits to the marinate, ensuring they are well-coated. Give it a minimum of fifteen minutes to marinate.
- Preheat the grill or grill pan to medium-high heat.
- Thread the marinating chicken cubes onto skewers.
- Grill the skewers for 5-6 minutes per side or until the chicken is cooked through and has grill marks.
- When serving, top with fresh parsley and lemon wedges.

Nutritional Values (per serving):

Calories: Approximately 180, Protein: 25g, Fat: 7g, Carbohydrates: 2g Fiber: 0.5g

Health Benefits:

1) Chicken offers a lean amount of energy.
2) Olive oil adds heart-healthy monounsaturated fats.

3) Lemon adds a delicious taste without extra calories.

4) Black pepper, thyme, and garlic powder improve taste without adding excessive salt.

Honey Mustard Chicken Salad

Preparation Time: 15 minutes

Cooking Time: 15 minutes

Servings: 4

Ingredients:

For Grilled Chicken:

- lbs boneless, skinless chicken breasts
- 2 tablespoons olive oil
- Salt and pepper to taste
- For Salad:

- Mixed salad greens
- Cherry tomatoes, split
- Cucumber, sliced
- Red onion, thinly sliced
- 1/4 cup crumbled feta (optional)
- For Honey Mustard Dressing:
- 3 tablespoons Dijon mustard
- 2 tablespoons honey
- 2 tablespoons olive oil
- 1 tablespoon apple cider vinegar
- Salt and pepper to taste

Instructions:

For Grilled Chicken:

- Preheat the grill or grill pan to medium-high heat.
- Add salt and pepper to the chicken breasts after brushing them with olive oil.

- Grill the chicken for 6-8 minutes per side or until it hits an internal temperature of 165°F (74°C). Before cutting, let it rest for a few minutes.

For Salad:

- In a big bowl, blend mixed salad leaves, cherry tomatoes, cucumber, and red onion.
- Top the salad with sliced grilled chicken. Add chopped feta cheese if wanted.
- For Honey Mustard Dressing:
- cheese
- In a small bowl, mix together Dijon mustard, honey, olive oil, apple cider vinegar, salt, and pepper.
- Drizzle the honey mustard sauce over the salad and toss gently to coat.

Nutritional Values (per serving):

Calories: Approximately 300,

Protein: 25g, Fat: 15g,

Carbohydrates: 15g, Fiber: 3g

Health Benefits:

1. Chicken gives lean energy.
2. Mixed salad leaves, peppers, and onion offer important nutrients and fiber.
3. Honey mustard sauce adds a sweet and tangy taste without extra calories.
4. Olive oil adds heart-healthy monounsaturated fats.

Teriyaki Chicken Stir-Fry

Preparation Time: 15 minutes

Cooking Time: 15 minutes

Servings: 4

Ingredients:

- o pounds of finely sliced, skinless, boneless chicken breasts
- 2 tablespoons soy sauce (low-sodium)
- 2 tablespoons teriyaki sauce
- 1 tablespoon hoisin sauce
- 1 tablespoon rice vinegar
- 1 tablespoon sesame oil
- 2 tablespoons vegetable oil
- 1 red bell pepper, finely sliced
- 1 yellow bell pepper, finely sliced
- 1 cup snap peas, ends cut
- 1 carrot, julienned
- 2 cloves garlic, minced
- 1 teaspoon fresh ginger, grated
- Cooked brown rice or quinoa for serving
- Sesame seeds and green onions for garnish

Instructions:

- In a bowl, mix soy sauce, teriyaki sauce, hoisin sauce, and rice vinegar to make the marinate.
- Marinate the sliced chicken in the mixture for at least 10 minutes.
- Heat vegetable oil in a wok or big pan over high heat.
- Stir-fry the marinating chicken until fully cooked and golden brown. Remove from the wok and set away.
- In the same pan, add sesame oil and stir-fry garlic and ginger until fragrant.
- Add bell peppers, snap peas, and julienned carrot. Stir-fry

until the veggies are tender-crisp.

- Return the cooked chicken to the pot and toss everything together to mix.
- Serve the teriyaki chicken stir-fry over cooked brown rice or quinoa.
- Add chopped green onions and sesame seeds as garnish.

Nutritional Values (per serving):

Calories: Approximately 350, Protein: 30g, Fat: 12g, Carbohydrates: 25g, Fiber: 5g

Health Benefits:

1. Chicken offers a lean amount of energy.
2. Colorful veggies offer a range of vitamins and minerals.
3. Teriyaki sauce adds taste without extra calories.
4. Sesame oil and seeds add healthy fats and a nutty taste.

BBQ Chicken Lettuce Wraps

Preparation Time: 15 minutes

Cooking Time: 15 minutes

Servings: 4

- **Ingredients:**
  - lbs boneless, skinless chicken breasts, cooked and shredded
- 1 cup barbecue sauce (choose a low-sugar or sugar-free choice)
- 1 tablespoon olive oil
- 1 red onion, finely chopped
- 1 bell pepper (any color), finely diced
- 2 cloves garlic, minced
- 1 teaspoon smoked pepper

- 1 teaspoon cumin
- Salt and pepper to taste
- Iceberg or butter lettuce leaves, for wrapping
- Optional toppings: Shredded cabbage, shredded carrots, sliced green onions, cilantro, lime wedges

Instructions:

- Lightly warm up some olive oil in a pan.
- Add diced red onion and bell pepper. Sauté until softened.
- Add chopped garlic, smoked paprika, and cumin. Sauté for an extra minute.
- Add chopped chicken to the pan and pour in BBQ sauce. Mix well to coat the chicken evenly. Cook until warm through.
- Season with salt and pepper to taste.
- Spoon the BBQ chicken mixture onto individual lettuce leaves.
- Top with extra additions like shredded cabbage, shredded carrots, sliced green onions, cilantro, and a squeeze of lime.
- Serve the BBQ chicken lettuce wraps instantly.

Nutritional Values (per serving):

Calories: Approximately 250, Protein: 25g, Fat: 7g, Carbohydrates: 20g, Fiber: 3g

Health Benefits:

1. Chicken offers a lean amount of energy.
2. Vegetables add important vitamins and minerals.

3. Choosing a low-sugar or sugar-free barbecue sauce lowers extra sugars.

4. Lettuce wraps offer a lighter option to standard wraps or tacos.

Buffalo Chicken Lettuce Wraps

Preparation Time: 15 minutes

Cooking Time: 15 minutes

Servings: 4

Ingredients:

- lbs boneless, skinless chicken breasts, cooked and shredded
- 1/2 cup buffalo sauce (choose a low-sugar or sugar-free version)
- 2 cups Greek yogurt or sour cream
- 1 tablespoon olive oil
- 1 celery stalk, finely chopped
- 1 carrot, shredded
- 1/4 cup blue cheese, crumbled
- Salt and pepper to taste
- Iceberg or butter lettuce leaves, for wrapping
- Optional toppings: Ranch sauce, sliced green onions, fresh parsley

Instructions:

- In a bowl, mix shredded chicken with buffalo sauce and Greek yogurt (or sour cream).
- Lightly warm up some olive oil in a pan.
- Add celery and chopped carrot to the pan. Sauté until softened.

- Add the buffalo chicken mixture to the pan and cook until warm through.
- Season with salt and pepper to taste.
- Spoon the spicy chicken filling onto individual lettuce leaves.
- Top with crumbled blue cheese and extra toppings like ranch dressing, sliced green onions, and fresh parsley.
- Serve the Buffalo Chicken Lettuce Wraps instantly.

Nutritional Values (per serving):

Calories: Approximately 280,
Protein: 30g, Fat: 12g,
Carbohydrates: 6g, Fiber: 2g

Health Benefits:

1. Chicken offers a lean amount of energy.
2. Vegetables add important vitamins and minerals.
3. Using Greek yogurt or sour cream offers a creamy texture with less fat.
4. Lettuce wraps provide a low-carb alternative to traditional wraps.

Mediterranean Grilled Chicken

Preparation Time: 15 minutes (plus marination time)

Cooking Time: 15 minutes

Servings: 4

Ingredients:

- lbs boneless, skinless chicken breasts
- 1/4 cup olive oil
- 2 tablespoons lemon juice
- 3 garlic cloves, chopped up

- 1 teaspoon dried oregano
- 1 teaspoon dried thyme
- 1 teaspoon crushed cumin
- Salt and pepper to taste
- Cherry tomatoes, for garnish
- Kalamata olives, for garnish
- Feta cheese, broken, for garnish
- Fresh parsley, chopped, for garnish

Instructions:

- In a bowl, mix together olive oil, lemon juice, chopped garlic, dried oregano, dried thyme, ground cumin, salt, and pepper to make the marinate.
- Place chicken breasts in a sealed plastic bag or small dish. Pour the sauce over the chicken, ensuring it's well-coated. Marinate in the refrigerator for at least 30 minutes, or ideally, a few hours.
- Preheat the grill to medium-high heat.
- Grill the chicken for 6-8 minutes per side or until it hits an internal temperature of 165°F (74°C) and has grill marks.
- Garnish with cherry tomatoes, Kalamata olives, crumbled feta cheese, and chopped fresh parsley.
- Serve the Mediterranean Grilled Chicken with your choice of sides, such as rice or a Greek salad.

Nutritional Values (per serving):

Calories: Approximately 300, Protein: 30g, Fat: 15g

Carbohydrates: 4g, Fiber: 1g

Health Benefits:

1. Chicken offers a lean amount of energy.
2. Olive oil adds heart-healthy monounsaturated fats.
3. Herbs and spices add taste without extra calories.
4. Mediterranean foods like tomatoes, olives, and feta offer a mix of nutrients.

Lime Cilantro Chicken

Preparation Time: 15 minutes (plus marination time)

Cooking Time: 15 minutes

Servings: 4

Ingredients:

- lbs boneless, skinless chicken breasts
- Zest and juice of 2 limes
- 1/4 cup olive oil
- 3 garlic cloves, chopped up
- 1 teaspoon crushed cumin
- 1 teaspoon pepper spice
- 1 teaspoon paprika
- Salt and pepper to taste
- Fresh cilantro, chopped, for garnish
- Lime wedges, for serving

Instructions:

- In a bowl, mix lime zest, lime juice, olive oil, chopped garlic, ground cumin, chili powder, paprika, salt, and pepper to make the marinate.
- Place chicken breasts in a sealed plastic bag or small dish. Pour the sauce over the

chicken, ensuring it's well-coated. Marinate in the refrigerator for at least 30 minutes, or ideally, a few hours.

- Preheat the grill to medium-high heat.
- Grill the chicken for 6-8 minutes per side or until it hits an internal temperature of 165°F (74°C) and has grill marks.
- Add fresh cilantro as a garnish and serve with lime wedges.
- Optionally, slice the grilled chicken and serve over a bed of rice or salad.

Nutritional Values (per serving):

Calories: Approximately 250, Protein: 30g, Fat: 12g, Carbohydrates: 2g, Fiber: 0.5g

Health Benefits:

1. Chicken offers a lean amount of energy.
2. Olive oil adds heart-healthy monounsaturated fats.
3. Lime adds a spicy taste without extra calories.
4. Cumin, pepper powder, and paprika improve taste without excessive salt.

Chicken and Veggie Skillet

Preparation Time: 15 minutes

Cooking Time: 20 minutes

Servings: 4

Ingredients:

- One and a half pounds of skinless, boneless chicken

breasts, sliced into small pieces

- 2 tablespoons olive oil
- 1 onion, finely sliced
- 2 bell peppers (any color), thinly sliced
- 1 zucchini, chopped
- 1 cup cherry tomatoes, sliced
- 3 garlic cloves, chopped up
- 1 teaspoon dried oregano
- 1 teaspoon dried basil
- Salt and pepper to taste
- Fresh parsley, chopped, for garnish

Instructions:

- In a large pan set over medium-high heat, warm the olive oil.
- Add chicken pieces and cook until browned on all sides and cooked through. Take out and put aside the chicken from the pan.
- If necessary, add a little more olive oil to the same pan.
- Add chopped onion, bell peppers, and zucchini. Sauté until veggies are tender-crisp.
- Add the minced garlic and continue cooking for one more minute.
- Return the cooked chicken to the pan.
- Toss in cherry tomatoes, dried oregano, dried basil, salt, and pepper. Cook for a few more minutes until tomatoes are slightly softened.
- Garnish with fresh parsley before serving.

Nutritional Values (per serving):

Calories: Approximately 300,
Protein: 30g, Fat: 10g,
Carbohydrates: 15g, Fiber: 4g

Health Benefits:

1. Chicken offers a lean amount of energy.
2. A number of colored veggies offer a range of vitamins and minerals.
3. Olive oil adds heart-healthy monounsaturated fats.
4. Herbs add taste without extra

Cranberry Balsamic Chicken

Preparation Time: 15 minutes (plus marination time)

Cooking Time: 25 minutes

Servings: 4

Ingredients:

- lbs boneless, skinless chicken breasts
- 1/2 cup cranberry sauce (ideally with no extra sugar)
- 1/4 cup balsamic vinegar
- 2 tablespoons olive oil
- 2 tablespoons soy sauce (low-sodium)
- 2 cloves garlic, minced
- 1 teaspoon dried rosemary
- Salt and pepper to taste
- Fresh cherries, for decoration (optional)
- Fresh parsley, chopped, for garnish

Instructions:

- In a bowl, mix together cranberry sauce, balsamic vinegar, olive oil, soy sauce, chopped garlic, dried

- rosemary, salt, and pepper to make the marinate.
- Place chicken breasts in a sealed plastic bag or small dish. Pour the sauce over the chicken, ensuring it's well-coated. Marinate in the refrigerator for at least 30 minutes, or ideally, a few hours.
- Preheat the oven to 375°F (190°C).
- Transfer the prepared chicken and sauce to a baking dish.
- Bake for 20-25 minutes or until the chicken is cooked through and no longer pink in the middle.
- Garnish with fresh cherries and chopped parsley before serving.

Nutritional Values (per serving):

Calories: Approximately 300, Protein: 30g, Fat: 10g, Carbohydrates: 20g, Fiber: 1.5g

Health Benefits:

1. Chicken offers a lean amount of energy.
2. Cranberries offer vitamins and possible health benefits.
3. Balsamic vinegar adds taste without extra calories.
4. This recipe is pretty low in added sugars if using a no-added-sugar cranberry sauce.

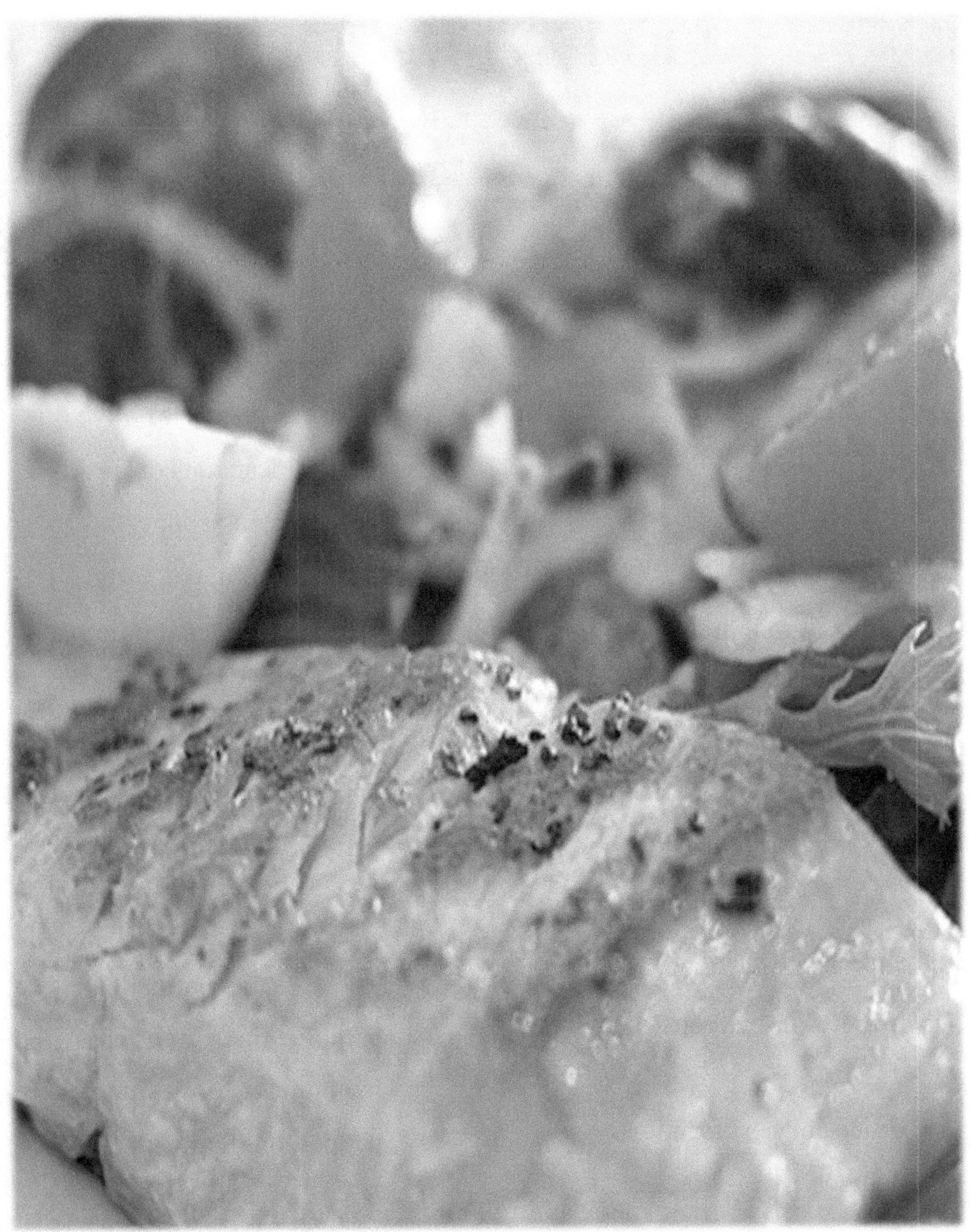

<u>**Chicken thighs with lemon pepper grilling:**</u>

Preparation Time: 10 minutes

(One hour of marinating time is optional.)

Cooking Time: 20 minutes

Servings: 4

Ingredients:

- Eight skin-on, bone-in chicken thighs
- Juice and zest from two lemons
- Three teaspoons of olive oil
- Two tablespoons of freshly ground black pepper
- one tsp powdered garlic
- One tsp powdered onion
- A single tsp of dried thyme
- Add salt to taste.
- Chopped fresh parsley (for garnish)

Instructions:

- To make the marinade, combine the lemon zest, lemon juice, olive oil, black pepper, onion powder, garlic powder, dried thyme, and salt in a bowl.

- Pour half of the marinade over the chicken thighs in a shallow dish or big resealable plastic bag. Keep the remaining half aside for basting.
- To enable the flavors to mingle, marinate the chicken for at least an hour in the fridge.
- Set the grill's temperature to medium-high.
- Take the chicken out of the marinade and throw away any leftover marinade.
- Baste the chicken thighs with the marinade that was set aside while grilling them for 8 to 10 minutes on each side, or until they are cooked through.
- Make sure the inside temperature reaches 74°C, or 165°F.
- Add some freshly cut parsley on top before serving.

Nutritional Value (Per servings):

(Note: Depending on certain components and portion proportions, nutritional values may change.)

Around 320 calories per serving., 25g of protein, 2 grams of carbohydrates, 22g of fat, Fiber: 0 grams

Health Benefits:

1. Protein-rich chicken thighs are a great option.
2. Lemon provides vitamin C and a tangy taste.

3. One source of good monounsaturated fats is olive oil.

4. Thyme and black pepper enhance flavor and antioxidants without adding extra calories.

Skewers of turkey and veggie meatballs:

Preparation Time: 20 minutes

Cooking Time: 15 minutes

Servings:4

Ingredients:

- One pound of ground turkey
- Half a cup of panko or whole wheat breadcrumbs
- 1/4 cup of Parmesan cheese, grated
- One egg
- two minced garlic cloves
- One tsp of dehydrated oregano
- To taste, add salt and pepper.
- One sliced zucchini
- One bell pepper, chopped into bits, any color
- One red onion, sliced into pieces
- rosy tomatoes
- Olive oil (to clean with)
- Metal or wood skewers

Instructions:

- Turn the heat up to medium-high on the grill or grill pan.
- Ground turkey, breadcrumbs, Parmesan cheese, egg, dried oregano, minced garlic, salt, and pepper should all be combined in a bowl. Blend until well blended.

- Shape the blend into little meatballs.
- Cherry tomatoes, bell pepper, red onion, and zucchini pieces are threaded onto skewers in succession with the meatballs.
- Apply some olive oil to the skewers.
- Turn the skewers once or twice while grilling them for approximately 12 to 15 minutes, or until the veggies are soft and browned and the meatballs are cooked through.
- Make sure the turkey meatballs are cooked through to an internal temperature of 165°F (74°C).
- Serve with tzatziki or your other dipping sauce, if desired.

Nutritional Value (Per servings):

(Note: Depending on certain components and portion proportions, nutritional values may change.)

Around 250 calories per serving., 20g of protein, 15g of carbohydrates, 10g of fat, 3g of fiber

Health Benefits:

1. Turkey is a low-fat protein source.
2. Vegetables provide fiber, vitamins, and minerals.
3. Monounsaturated fats, found in olive oil, are good for you.
4. This recipe is a healthy, well-balanced choice for a delightful, light supper.

<u>**Baked Chicken Tenders with Garlic and Parmesan:**</u>

Preparation Time: 15 minutes.

Cooking Time: 15 minutes

Servings:4

Ingredients:

- One-pound chicken tenders
- One cup of panko or whole wheat breadcrumbs
- Grated Parmesan cheese, half a cup
- two tsp powdered garlic
- One tsp of dehydrated oregano
- To taste, add salt and pepper.
- Half a cup of flour, whole wheat or all-purpose
- two beaten eggs
- Olive oil or cooking spray (for coating)

Instructions:

- Set oven temperature to 400°F, or 200°C. Grease a baking sheet gently or line it with parchment paper.
- Mix breadcrumbs, grated Parmesan cheese, dried oregano, garlic powder, salt, and pepper in a shallow dish. Blend well.
- Transfer flour to a another shallow dish.
- After dredging each chicken tender in flour, shake off any excess.
- After flouring the chicken, dip it into the beaten eggs.
- Apply the breadcrumb mixture to the chicken, pressing it firmly to stick to the tenders.
- Arrange the coated chicken tenders onto the baking sheet that has been ready.

- Apply a little layer of cooking spray or olive oil to the tenders' tops.
- Bake the chicken for 12 to 15 minutes, or until it's cooked through and has a golden brown color, in a preheated oven.
- Serve with your preferred dipping sauce or a side of marinara sauce, if desired.

Nutritional Value (Per servings):

(Note: Depending on certain components and portion proportions, nutritional values may change.)

Around 250 calories per serving., 30g of protein, 15g of carbohydrates, 8g of fat, 2g of fiber

Health Benefits:

1. Reduced total fat content because baked rather than fried.
2. Lean protein may be found in abundance in chicken tenders.
3. Flavor is added with parmesan cheese without adding too many calories.
4. Oregano and garlic provide flavor and may have health advantages.

Asian Lettuce Wraps with Turkey:

Preparation Time: 15 minutes.

Cooking Time: 15 minutes

Servings:4

Ingredients:

- One pound of ground turkey

- One tablespoon of sesame oil

- One onion, chopped finely

- two minced garlic cloves

- One tablespoon of grated ginger

- 1/4 cup low-sodium soy sauce

- Two tsp of hoisin sauce.

- One-tspn rice vinegar

- One tablespoon of optional Sriracha sauce

- One cup of chopped water chestnuts

- chop half a cup of green onions

- 1/4 cup finely chopped fresh cilantro

- Leaves of iceberg or butter lettuce (to wrap)

Instructions:

- Sesame oil should be heated over medium heat in a big skillet.

- To the skillet, add the minced garlic, grated ginger, and chopped onion. Add the onion and sauté until it's soft.

- Using a spoon, break up the ground turkey as it cooks until it becomes brown in the pan.

- Combine the rice vinegar, soy sauce, hoisin sauce, and Sriracha (if using) in a bowl. Cover the turkey mixture with the sauce.

- Add chopped fresh cilantro, green onions, and water chestnuts. Cook for a further two to three minutes, or until well heated.

- To make lettuce wraps, spoon the turkey mixture over the leaves.

- Garnish with more green onions and cilantro, if desired.

- Serve right away.

Nutritional Value (Per servings):

(Note: Depending on certain components and portion proportions, nutritional values may change.)

Around 250 calories per serving., 20g of protein, 15g of carbohydrates, 12g of fat, 3g of fiber

Health Benefits:

1. Turkey is a low-fat protein source.
2. Healthy lipids and a nutty taste are added by sesame oil.
3. Water chestnuts have a delightful texture and crunch.
4. Wraps made of lettuce are a low-carb substitute for regular wraps.

Garlic and Rosemary Grilled Lamb Chops:

Preparation Time: 15 minutes.

One hour of marinating time is optional.

Cooking Time: 10 minutes

Servings:4

Ingredients:

- Eight chops of lamb
- Three teaspoons of olive oil
- three minced garlic cloves
- Two teaspoons of freshly chopped rosemary
- One tsp Dijon mustard
- To taste, add salt and pepper.
- slices of lemon (for serving)
- **Instructions:**

- To make the marinade, combine olive oil, minced garlic, finely chopped fresh rosemary, Dijon mustard, salt, and pepper in a bowl.
- Pour the marinade over the lamb chops and place them in a shallow dish. If you have time, marinate in the fridge for at least an hour.
- Set the grill's temperature to medium-high.
- Take the lamb chops out of the marinade and throw away any leftover marinade.
- For medium-rare, grill the lamb chops for 4–5 minutes on each side, modifying the cooking time according to your preferred level of doneness.
- Make sure the lamb is cooked through at 145°F (63°C), 160°F (71°C), or 170°F (77°C) for medium-rare, medium, or well-done.
- Optional: Before serving, squeeze some lemon juice over the cooked lamb chops.

Nutritional Value (Per servings):

(Note: Depending on certain components and portion proportions, nutritional values may change.)

Around 300 calories per serving., 25g of protein, 0g of carbohydrates 22g of fat, Fiber: 0 grams

Health Benefits:

1. One of the best sources of high-quality protein is lamb.
2. Healthy monounsaturated fats are added by the olive oil in the marinade.

3. In addition to adding taste, garlic and rosemary may provide health advantages.

4. This is a tasty, high-protein alternative for a grilled supper.

Salmon with Teriyaki Glaze:

Preparation Time: 10 minutes

Allow 30 minutes for marinating (optional).

Cooking Time: 15 minutes

Servings: 4

Ingredients:

- Four fillets of salmon
- Half a cup of soy sauce (low sodium)
- three tsp honey
- two tsp of rice vinegar
- One tablespoon of sesame oil
- two minced garlic cloves
- one tsp finely grated ginger
- One tablespoon cornstarch (to thicken, if desired)
- Green onions with sesame seeds (as a garnish)

Instructions:

- To make the teriyaki sauce, combine the soy sauce, honey, rice vinegar, sesame oil, chopped garlic, and grated ginger in a bowl.
- Transfer half of the teriyaki sauce to a shallow dish and cover the salmon fillets with it. Keep the remaining half aside for dishing and basting.
- If desired, marinate the salmon for at least half an hour in the fridge.
- Set oven temperature to 400°F, or 200°C.

- Grease a baking sheet gently or line it with parchment paper.
- Arrange the marinated salmon fillets onto the baking sheet that has been ready.
- Bake the salmon for 12 to 15 minutes, or until it is cooked through and flake readily with a fork, in an oven that has been warmed.
- Optional: Reheat the set-aside teriyaki sauce in a small pot over medium heat. If desired, thin the sauce by adding a slurry made of cornstarch and a little amount of water to the sauce.
- In the last minutes of baking, brush the salmon with the thickened teriyaki sauce.
- Before serving, garnish with chopped green onions and sesame seeds.

Nutritional Value (Per servings):

(Note: Depending on certain components and portion proportions, nutritional values may change.)

Around 350 calories per serving., 25g of protein, 20g of carbohydrates, 18g of fat, Fiber: 0 grams

Health Benefits:

1. For heart health, omega-3 fatty acids are abundant in salmon.
2. Flavor is added with teriyaki sauce without adding too many calories.

3. Garlic and ginger improve flavor and may be good for your health.

4. This is a tasty and healthy seafood meal to have for supper.

Tzatziki Sauced Mediterranean Turkey Burgers:

Preparation Time: 15 minutes.

Cooking Time: 15 minutes

Servings: 4

Ingredients:

Regarding Turkcy Burgcrs:

- One pound of ground turkey
- Half a cup of panko or whole wheat breadcrumbs
- 1/4 cup of crumbled feta cheese
- 1/4 cup finely chopped Kalamata olives
- 1/4 cup chopped sun-dried tomatoes
- two minced garlic cloves
- One tsp of dehydrated oregano
- To taste, add salt and pepper.
- Castor oil (to grill)

Regarding Tzatziki Sauce:

- One cup of Greek yogurt
- half of a cucumber, drained and shredded
- Two teaspoons of freshly chopped dill
- One tablespoon of lemon juice
- one minced garlic clove
- To taste, add salt and pepper.

Instructions:

Regarding Turkey Burgers:

- Ground turkey, breadcrumbs, crumbled feta cheese, chopped sun-dried tomatoes, chopped Kalamata olives, minced garlic, dried oregano, salt, and pepper should all be combined in a dish. Blend until well blended.
- Create four burger patties out of the mixture.
- Turn the heat up to medium-high on the grill or grill pan.
- Burgers should be cooked through after grilling for 6 to 8 minutes on each side, brushed with olive oil.
- Make sure the turkey burgers are cooked through to an internal temperature of 165°F (74°C).

Regarding Tzatziki Sauce:

- Greek yogurt, grated and drained cucumber, chopped fresh dill, lemon juice, minced garlic, salt, and pepper should all be combined in a bowl.
- The tzatziki sauce should be kept chilled until needed.

Nutritional Value (Per servings):

(Note: Depending on certain components and portion proportions, nutritional values may change.)

About 300 calories are included in each serving (burger plus sauce), 25g of protein, 15g of carbohydrates, 15g of fat, 2g of fiber

Health Benefits:

- Lean protein is available from turkey.
- Antioxidants and taste are added by Mediterranean ingredients.
- Greek yogurt has probiotics, and tzatziki sauce has a cool flavor.
- This recipe is a more healthful take on classic beef burgers.

Dill and Lemon Baked Cod:

Preparation Time: 10 minutes

Allow 30 minutes for marinating (optional).

Cooking Time: 15 minutes

Servings: 4

Ingredients:

- Four fillets of cod
- One lemon's juice and zest
- Two tsp olive oil
- Two teaspoons of freshly chopped dill
- two minced garlic cloves
- To taste, add salt and pepper.
- Slices of lemon (as a garnish)

Instructions:

- To make the marinade, combine the lemon zest, lemon juice, olive oil, minced garlic, chopped fresh dill, salt, and pepper in a bowl.
- Transfer half of the marinade to a shallow dish and cover the fish fillets with it. Keep the remaining half aside for dishing and basting.
- If desired, marinate the fish for at least half an hour in the fridge.

- Set oven temperature to 400°F, or 200°C.
- Grease a baking sheet gently or line it with parchment paper.
- The cod fillets should be marinated and placed on the ready baking pan.
- Bake the fish for 12 to 15 minutes in a preheated oven, or until it is cooked through and flake easily with a fork.
- Optional: During the last few minutes of baking, baste the cod with the marinade that was set aside.
- Before serving, garnish with slices of lemon.

Nutritional Value (Per servings):

(Note: Depending on certain components and portion proportions, nutritional values may change.)

Around 200 calories per serving., 25g of protein, 2 grams of carbohydrates, 10g of fat, Fiber: 0 grams

Health Benefits:

1. Cod is low in calories and a lean protein source.
2. Lemon provides vitamin C and a crisp citrus taste.
3. Monounsaturated fats, found in olive oil, are good for you.
4. Dill adds a distinct flavor and perhaps health advantages.

Cilantro-Lime Chicken Kebabs:

Preparation Time: 15 minutes.

One hour is needed for marinating.

Cooking Time: 10 minutes

Servings: 4

Ingredients:

- One and a half pounds of skinless, boneless cubed chicken breasts
- Juice and zest from two limes
- Two tsp olive oil
- One tablespoon of powdered chilies
- One teaspoon of cumin
- one tsp powdered garlic
- One tsp powdered onion
- To taste, add salt and pepper.
- Finely chopped fresh cilantro (for garnish)
- slices of lime (for serving)

Instructions:

- To make the marinade, combine the lime zest, lime juice, olive oil, cumin, chili powder, onion powder, garlic powder, salt, and pepper in a bowl.
- Toss the chicken cubes in the basin to ensure that they are equally covered with marinade.
- The chicken should marinate in the bowl for at least an hour. Cover and refrigerate.
- Turn the heat up to medium-high on the grill or grill pan.
- Put marinated chunks of chicken on skewers.
- Cook the chicken on the skewers for approximately 5 minutes on each side, or until it is cooked through and has grill marks.

- Make sure the chicken achieves an internal temperature of 165°F or 74°C.
- Optional: Serve with lime wedges and sprinkle with freshly chopped cilantro.

Nutritional Value (Per servings):

(Note: Depending on certain components and portion proportions, nutritional values may change.)

Around 250 calories per serving., 0g of protein, 5g of carbohydrates, 12g of fat, 1g of fiber

Health Benefits:

One lean protein source is chicken.

Lime provides vitamin C and a tangy taste.

The marinade's olive oil provides beneficial monounsaturated fats.

This dish may be included in a balanced diet since it is low in carbs.

Pork Tenderloin with a Balsamic Glaze:

Preparation Time: 10 minutes

One hour of marinating time is optional.

Cooking Time: 20 minutes

Servings: 4

Ingredients:

- Two one-pound tenderloins of pork
- Balsamic vinegar, half a cup

- 1/4 cup of honey

- Two teaspoons of low-sodium soy sauce

- two minced garlic cloves

- One tsp Dijon mustard

- To taste, add salt and pepper.

- Finely chopped fresh rosemary (for garnish)

Instructions:

- To make the marinade, combine the balsamic vinegar, honey, soy sauce, minced garlic, Dijon mustard, salt, and pepper in a bowl.

- Transfer half of the marinade to a shallow dish and cover the pork tenderloins with it. Keep the remaining half aside for basting.

- Allow the flavors to seep into the pork by marinating it for at least an hour in the fridge.

- Set oven temperature to 400°F, or 200°C.

- Take the pork tenderloins out of the marinade and throw away any leftover marinade.

- Using parchment paper or a baking dish that has been oiled, place the pork on the baking sheet.

- Roast for approximately 20 minutes, or until the internal temperature reaches 145°F (63°C), in the preheated oven.

- During the last ten minutes of cooking, baste the pork with the marinade that was set aside.

- Optional: Before serving, sprinkle some freshly chopped rosemary over top.

Nutritional Value (Per servings):

(Note: Depending on certain components and portion proportions, nutritional values may change.)

Around 250 calories per serving, 25g of protein, 20g of carbohydrates, 8g of fat, Fiber: 0 grams

Health Benefits:

1. Lean protein may be found in pork tenderloin.
2. Without adding additional calories, balsamic vinegar gives a sweet and tart taste.
3. Antioxidants and natural sweetness are provided by honey.
4. This dish may be included in a balanced diet and is a wonderful source of protein.

Cajun Skillet with Sausage and Shrimp:

Preparation Time: 15 minutes.

Cooking Time: 15 minutes

Servings: 4

Ingredients:

- One pound of big, peeled and deveined shrimp
- 1 pound of sliced smoked sausage
- One sliced bell pepper
- One sliced onion
- three minced garlic cloves
- One 14-oz can of chopped, drained tomatoes
- Two tsp of Cajun spice
- One tsp of paprika
- Half a teaspoon of thyme
- To taste, add salt and pepper.

- chopped green onions (for garnish)
- Prepared rice (to be served)

Instructions:

- Heat the olive oil in a big pan over medium-high heat.
- Cook the sausage slices in the pan until they are browned.
- To the pan, add the minced garlic, onion, and bell pepper. Make sure that the veggies are cooked until they are soft.
- When the shrimp are pink and opaque, add them to the skillet and simmer.
- Add the diced tomatoes, paprika, thyme, Cajun spice, salt, and pepper and stir. Cook for a further two to three minutes.
- Serve over cooked rice if desired.
- Before serving, sprinkle some chopped green onions on top.

Nutritional Value (Per servings):

(Note: Depending on certain components and portion proportions, nutritional values may change.)

Around 400 calories per serving., 25g of protein, 15g of carbohydrates, 25g of fat, 2g of fiber

Health Benefits:

1. Lean protein is found in shrimp.
2. The meal gains flavor and richness from the sausage.
3. Onions and bell peppers provide fiber and vitamins.
4. A tasty supper may be had quickly and satisfactorily with this skillet dish.

<u>**Shrimp with Lemon Garlic Butter:**</u>

Preparation Time: 10 minutes

Cooking Time: 10 minutes

Servings: 4

Ingredients:

- One pound of big, peeled and deveined shrimp
- Four tsp unsalted butter
- four minced garlic cloves
- One lemon's juice and zest
- One tsp of dehydrated oregano
- Half a teaspoon of optional red pepper flakes
- To taste, add salt and pepper.
- Chopped fresh parsley (for garnish)
- cooked rice or pasta (to serve)

Instructions:

- Melt butter in a big skillet over a medium heat.
- Garlic powder should be added to the pan and cooked until aromatic.
- When the shrimp are pink and opaque, add them to the skillet and simmer.
- Add the zest and juice of the lemon, dried oregano, salt, pepper, and red pepper flakes (if using). Cook for a further two to three minutes.
- Serve over cooked rice or pasta, if desired.
- Top with some freshly cut parsley just before serving.

Nutritional Value (Per Servings):

(Note: Depending on certain components and portion

proportions, nutritional values may change.)

Around 250 calories per serving., 25g of protein, 2 grams of carbohydrates, 15g of fat, Fiber: 0 grams

Health Benefits:

1. Lean protein is found in shrimp.
2. Oregano and garlic enhance taste and may have health advantages.
3. Lemon adds vitamin C and a crisp citrus flavor.
4. This dish may be included in a balanced diet since it is low in car

Cucumber Bites with Grilled Lemon Herb Chicken

Preparation Time: 20 minutes (including marination time)

Cooking Time: 15 minutes

Servings: 4

Ingredients:

- lbs boneless, skinless chicken breasts
- Two lemons' zest and juice
- 2 tablespoons olive oil
- 1 teaspoon dried thyme
- 1 teaspoon dried rosemary
- 1 teaspoon garlic powder
- Salt and pepper to taste
- 2 large cucumbers, sliced into rounds
- Cherry tomatoes, sliced, for garnish
- Fresh parsley, chopped, for garnish

Instructions:

- In a bowl, mix olive oil, lemon zest, lemon juice, dried thyme, dried rosemary, garlic powder, salt, and pepper to make the marinade.

- Place chicken breasts in a sealed plastic bag or small dish. Pour the sauce over the chicken, ensuring it's well-coated. Marinate in the refrigerator for at least 30 minutes, or ideally, a few hours.
- Preheat the grill to medium-high heat.
- Grill the chicken for 6-8 minutes per side or until it hits an internal temperature of 165°F (74°C) and has grill marks.
- Let the chicken rest for a few minutes, then slice it into thin pieces.
- Place cucumber circles on a serving plate.
- Top each cucumber round with a slice of grilled lemon herb chicken.
- Garnish with cherry tomato halves and chopped fresh parsley.

Nutritional Values (per serving):

Calories: Approximately 200,

Protein: 25g, Fat: 8g,

Carbohydrates: 5g, Fiber: 2g

Health Benefits:

1. Chicken offers a lean amount of energy.
2. Cucumbers add a refreshing crunch and hydration.
3. Lemon, thyme, and rosemary contribute flavor without excessive calories.
4. This recipe is low in carbohydrates and offers a light and satisfying appetizer.

Deviled Eggs

Preparation Time: 20 minutes

Cooking Time: 12 minutes

Servings: 6 (2 halves per serve)

Ingredients:

- 6 large eggs
- 2 tablespoons mayonnaise
- 1 teaspoon Dijon mustard
- 1 teaspoon white vinegar
- Salt and pepper to taste
- Paprika and fresh onions for decoration (optional)

Instructions:

- Place eggs in a single layer in a pot and cover with water. Bring to a boil, then reduce heat to a simmer and cook for 10-12 minutes.
- Remove eggs from hot water and place them in an ice water bath to cool.
- Peel and cut the eggs in half lengthwise after they have cooled.
- Remove the yolks with care and put them in a bowl. Mash the eggs with a fork.
- You can mix the beaten yolks with Dijon mustard, white vinegar, salt, and pepper. Mix until smooth and well mixed.
- Add the yolk mixture back to the egg whites with a spoon or a pipe.
- Garnish with paprika and fresh onions if wanted.

Nutritional Values (for a serving of two halves):

Calories: about 120, 6g of protein, Fat: 9g, Carbohydrates: 1g, Fiber: 0 grams

Health Benefits:

1. Eggs provide high-quality energy.
2. When used in moderation, mayonnaise makes things creamier without adding too many calories.
3. Mustard and vinegar add taste without extra fat.
4. This meal is low in sugars and makes for a protein-rich snack or starter.

Veggie Sticks with Hummus

Preparation Time: 15 minutes

Cooking Time: 0 minutes

Servings: 4

Ingredients:

- Assorted veggies (carrots, cucumber, bell peppers, cherry tomatoes)
- Hummus for dipping (store-bought or homemade)

Instructions:

- Wash and peel (if necessary) the veggies.
- Cut the carrots, onion, and bell peppers into stick forms.
- Arrange the veggie sticks on a serving plate.
- Serve with hummus for dipping.

Nutritional Values (per serving):

Calories: Approximately 100, Protein: 4g, Fat: 5g, Carbohydrates: 12g, Fiber: 4g

Health Benefits

1. Assorted veggies provide a range of vitamins and minerals.
2. Hummus offers plant-based nutrition and healthy fats.
3. This meal is low in calories and high in fiber, making it a healthy and delicious lunch.
4. Vegetables are rich in vitamins and add to general health.

Zucchini Chips

Preparation Time: 15 minutes

Cooking Time: 25 minutes

Servings: 4

Ingredients:

- 2 large zucchinis, thinly sliced
- 2 tablespoons olive oil
- 1/2 cup grated Parmesan cheese
- 1/2 cup breadcrumbs (preferred whole wheat)
- 1 teaspoon garlic powder
- 1 teaspoon dried oregano
- Salt and pepper to taste

Instructions:

- Preheat the oven to 425°F (220°C).
- In a bowl, mix olive oil, grated Parmesan, breadcrumbs, garlic powder, dried oregano, salt, and pepper.
- Dip each zucchini slice into the breadcrumb mixture, covering both sides.
- Place the covered zucchini slices on a baking sheet lined with parchment paper.

- Bake for 20-25 minutes or until the zucchini chips are golden brown and crunchy.
- To ensure the chips are ready to be served, it's important to allow them some time to cool down beforehand.

Nutritional Values (per serving):

Calories: about 120, Protein: 5g, Fat: 7g, Carbohydrates: 10g, Fiber: 2g

Health Benefits:

- Zucchini is a vegetable that is rich in vitamins and minerals and has very few calories.
- Olive oil gives heart-healthy monounsaturated fats.
- Parmesan cheese gives taste without extra calories.

- Baked, not fried, making these chips a healthy option to standard potato chips.

Greek Yogurt Dip

Preparation Time: 10 minutes

Cooking Time: 0 minutes

Servings: 6

Ingredients:

- 1 cup Greek yogurt (plain, whole-milk or low-fat)
- 1 tablespoon olive oil
- 1 tablespoon lemon juice
- 1 clove garlic, minced
- 1 teaspoon dried dill
- Salt and pepper to taste

Instructions:

- In a bowl, mix Greek yogurt, olive oil, lemon juice, chopped garlic, dried dill, salt, and pepper.
- Mix the items until well mixed.
- Adjust salt to taste.
- Refrigerate the dip for at least 30 minutes to allow the flavors to mix.
- Serve chilled with veggies, pita bread, or as a topping for grilled meats.

Nutritional Values (per serving):

Calories: Approximately 60, Protein: 5g, Fat: 4g, Carbohydrates: 2g, Sugar: 1g

Health Benefits:

1. Greek yogurt offers a great source of protein and probiotics.
2. Olive oil adds heart-healthy monounsaturated fats.
3. Lemon juice adds a delicious lemon taste.
4. Dill offers a rush of taste without extra calories.

Stuffed Mini Bell Peppers

Preparation Time: 20 minutes

Cooking Time: 15 minutes

Servings: 4-6 (2-3 peppers per dish)

Ingredients:

- 12-18 tiny bell peppers, split and seeds removed
- 1 cup cooked quinoa or rice

- 1 cup black beans, drained and washed
- 1 cup corn kernels (fresh or frozen)
- 1 cup chopped tomatoes
- 1/2 cup shredded cheese (cheddar or Mexican mix)
- 1 teaspoon crushed cumin
- 1 teaspoon pepper spice
- Salt and pepper to taste
- Fresh cilantro, chopped, for garnish

Instructions:

- Preheat the oven to 375°F (190°C).
- In a bowl, mix cooked quinoa or rice, black beans, corn, diced tomatoes, sliced cheese, ground cumin, chili powder, salt, and pepper.
- Stuff each small bell pepper half with the rice filling.
- On a baking sheet, arrange the filled peppers.
- Bake for 15 minutes or until the peppers are soft and the sauce is warm through.
- Garnish with fresh cilantro before serving.

Nutritional Values (per serve - 3 peppers)

Calories: Approximately 250, Protein: 10g, Fat: 6g, Carbohydrates: 40g, Fiber: 8g

Health Benefits:

1. Bell peppers provide a rich source of vitamins A and C.
2. Quinoa offers full protein and vital amino acids.
3. Black beans and corn add nutrients and extra energy.

4. This recipe is a well-balanced, meatless choice rich in nutrients.

5. Stuffed Mini Bell Peppers are a bright and delicious dish that serves as a filling snack or light meal. Enjoy the health benefits and lively taste of this delicious meal!

Fruit Salad Skewers

Preparation Time: 20 minutes

Cooking Time: 0 minutes

Servings: 4 (3-4 skewers per dish)

Ingredients:

- Assorted fruits (strawberries, pineapple chunks, grapes, melon bits, etc.)
- 1 tablespoon honey or maple syrup (optional)
- Fresh mint leaves for garnish

Instructions:

- Cut the vegetables into bite-sized pieces after washing and preparing.
- Thread the fruit pieces onto skewers, changing colors and types.
- Optionally, drizzle honey or maple syrup over the fruit sticks for extra sweetness.
- Garnish with fresh mint leaves.
- Serve directly or chill until ready to serve.

Nutritional Values (per serving):

Calories: Approximately 80, Protein: 1g, Fat: 0.5g, Carbohydrates: 20g, Fiber: 3g

Health Benefits:

1. Antioxidants, minerals, and vitamins abound in fruits.
2. Honey or maple syrup adds a touch of natural sweetness without excessive added sugars.
3. This recipe is low in calories and offers a cool and hydrating treat.
4. Fruit Salad Skewers provide a bright and healthy dessert or snack choice.

Cauliflower Popcorn

Preparation Time: 15 minutes

Cooking Time: 25 minutes

Servings: 4

Ingredients:

- 1 large cauliflower head, cut into bite-sized pieces
- 2 tablespoons olive oil
- 1 teaspoon garlic powder
- 1 teaspoon onion powder
- 1 teaspoon paprika
- Salt and pepper to taste
- Fresh parsley, chopped, for garnish (optional)
- Instructions:

- Preheat the oven to 425°F (220°C).
- In a large bowl, toss cauliflower pieces with olive oil, garlic powder, onion powder, paprika, salt, and pepper until well covered.
- Spread the seasoned broccoli on a baking sheet in a single layer.

- Roast for 25 minutes or until the cauliflower is golden brown and crispy.
- Garnish with chopped fresh parsley if wanted.
- Serve quickly.

Nutritional Values (per serving):

Calories: Approximately 100, Protein: 4g, Fat: 7g, Carbohydrates: 10g, Fiber: 4g

Health Benefits:

1. Cauliflower is a low-calorie food rich in vitamins and minerals.
2. Olive oil gives heart-healthy monounsaturated fats.
3. Garlic and onion powder add taste without extra calories.
4. This dish is a healthy alternative to traditional popcorn, giving a delicious crunch and spicy taste.

Tuna Cucumber Bites

Preparation Time: 15 minutes

Cooking Time: 0 minutes

Servings: 4

Ingredients

- Five-ounce can of drained tuna in water
- 1/4 cup mayonnaise
- 1 teaspoon Dijon mustard
- Salt and pepper to taste
- 2 cucumbers, sliced into rounds
- Cherry tomatoes, sliced, for garnish
- Fresh dill or parsley, chopped, for garnish

Instructions:

- In a bowl, mix drained tuna with mayonnaise and Dijon mustard. Season with salt and pepper to taste.
- Place cucumber circles on a serving plate.
- Spoon a small amount of the tuna mixture onto each cucumber round.
- Garnish with cherry tomato halves and chopped fresh dill or parsley.
- Serve quickly.

Nutritional Values (per serving):

Calories: Approximately 150, Protein: 10g, Fat: 10g, Carbohydrates: 5g, Fiber: 1.5g

Health Benefits:

1. Tuna offers a healthy form of protein and omega-3 fatty acids.
2. Cucumbers add a delicious crunch and moisture.
3. Mayonnaise and Dijon mustard add taste without extra calories.
4. This meal is low in calories and offers a light and filling snack.

Baked Buffalo Cauliflower Bites

Preparation Time: 15 minutes

Cooking Time: 25 minutes

Servings: 4

Ingredients:

- 1 large cauliflower head, cut into bite-sized pieces

- 1/2 cup flour (all-purpose or chickpea flour for a gluten-free choice)
- 1/2 cup milk (dairy or plant-based)
- 1 teaspoon garlic powder
- 1 teaspoon onion powder
- 1/2 cup buffalo sauce
- 2 tablespoons melted butter or olive oil
- Ranch or blue cheese dressing for dipping

Instructions:

- Preheat the oven to 450°F (230°C) and line a baking sheet with parchment paper.
- In a bowl, mix flour, milk, garlic powder, and onion powder to make a batter.
- Dip each cauliflower floret into the batter, ensuring it's well-coated, and place it on the baking sheet.
- Bake for 20 minutes or until the cauliflower is golden brown and crispy.
- In a different bowl, mix buffalo sauce and melted butter or olive oil.
- Toss the baked cauliflower in the buffalo sauce mixture until evenly coated.
- Return the coated cauliflower to the baking sheet and bake for an additional 5 minutes.
- Present with dips like blue cheese or ranch dressing.

Nutritional Values (per serving):

Calories: Approximately 150, Protein: 5g, Fat: 7g, Carbohydrates: 20g, Fiber: 4g

Health Benefits:

1. Cauliflower is a low-calorie food rich in vitamins and minerals.
2. Baking instead of frying lowers extra fats and calories.
3. Buffalo sauce adds taste without extra calories.
4. This dish offers a tasty and better alternative to standard buffalo wings

Apple Slices with Cinnamon

Preparation Time: 5 minutes

Cooking Time: 0 minutes

Servings: 2

Ingredients:

- 2 big apples, cored and sliced
- 1 teaspoon dried cinnamon

Instructions:

- Core and slice the apples into thin rounds or pieces.
- Arrange the apple slices on a plate or serving dish.
- Sprinkle ground cinnamon over the apple pieces.
- Gently toss the slices to ensure an even covering of cinnamon.
- Serve quickly.

Nutritional Values (per serving):

Calories: Approximately 100,

Protein: 0.5g, Fat: 0.3g,

Carbohydrates: 26g, Fiber: 5g

Health Benefits:

1. Vitamins, fiber, and antioxidants abound in apples.
2. Cinnamon gives taste without extra calories or sugar.
3. This meal is low in calories, making it a healthy and delicious snack.

4. The natural sweetness of apples can help curb sugar cravings.

Salsa and Baked Pita Chips

Preparation Time: 15 minutes

Cooking Time: 10 minutes

Servings: 4

Ingredients:

For Salsa:

- 4 medium tomatoes, diced
- 1/2 red onion, roughly chopped
- 1 jalapeño, seeds and diced
- 1/4 cup fresh cilantro, chopped
- 1 clove garlic, minced
- Juice of 1 lime
- Salt and pepper to taste

For Baked Pita Chips:

- 4 whole wheat pita bread rounds
- 2 tablespoons olive oil
- 1 teaspoon crushed cumin
- 1 teaspoon paprika
- Salt to taste

Instructions:

For Salsa:

- In a bowl, mix diced tomatoes, chopped red onion, jalapeño, cilantro, minced garlic, lime juice, salt, and pepper. Mix well.

- Refrigerate the salsa for at least 30 minutes to allow tastes to meld.

For Baked Pita Chips:

- Preheat the oven to 375°F (190°C).
- Brush each bread round with olive oil on both sides.
- In a small bowl, mix ground cumin, paprika, and salt.
- Sprinkle the spice combination over the oiled pita pieces.
- Cut each bread round into pieces and place them on a baking sheet.
- Bake for 8-10 minutes or until the pita chips are crisp and brown.

Nutritional Values (per serving):

Calories: Approximately 150, Protein: 3g, Fat: 7g, Carbohydrates: 20g, Fiber: 4g

Health Benefits:

1. Tomatoes provide vitamins, minerals, and water.
2. Whole wheat pita adds fiber and calories to the snack.
3. Olive oil adds heart-healthy monounsaturated fats.
4. This dish offers a delicious and tasty option to standard chips and salsa.

THE MEAL PLANNER

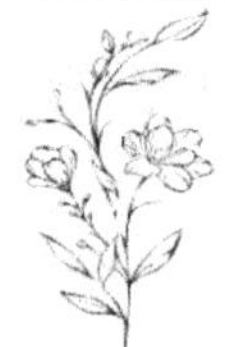

Date__________

	BREAKFAST	LUNCH	DINNER	SNACKS
MON				
TUE				
WED				
THU				
FRI				
SAT				
SUN				

Note

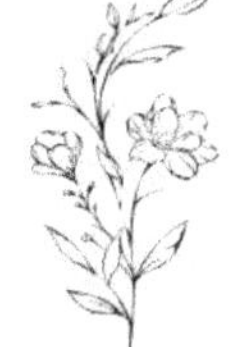
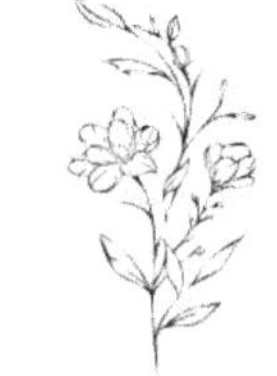

Zero Point Weekly Meal planner

for the week

Date __________

	BREAKFAST	LUNCH	DINNER	SNACKS
MON				
TUE				
WED				
THU				
FRI				
SAT				
SUN				

Note

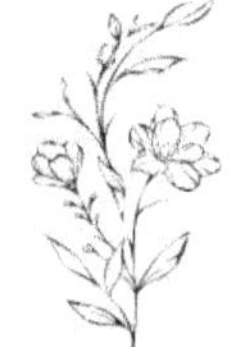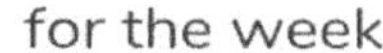

Zero Point Weekly Meal planner

for the week

Date___________

	BREAKFAST	LUNCH	DINNER	SNACKS
MON				
TUE				
WED				
THU				
FRI				
SAT				
SUN				

Note

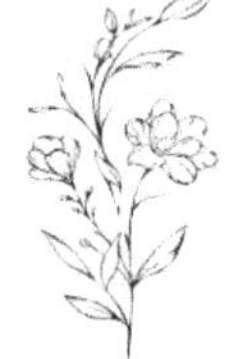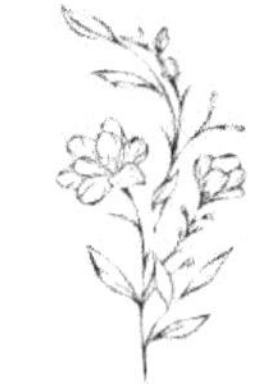

Zero Point Weekly Meal planner

for the week

Date__________

	BREAKFAST	LUNCH	DINNER	SNACKS
MON				
TUE				
WED				
THU				
FRI				
SAT				
SUN				

Note